dancing
with the stars

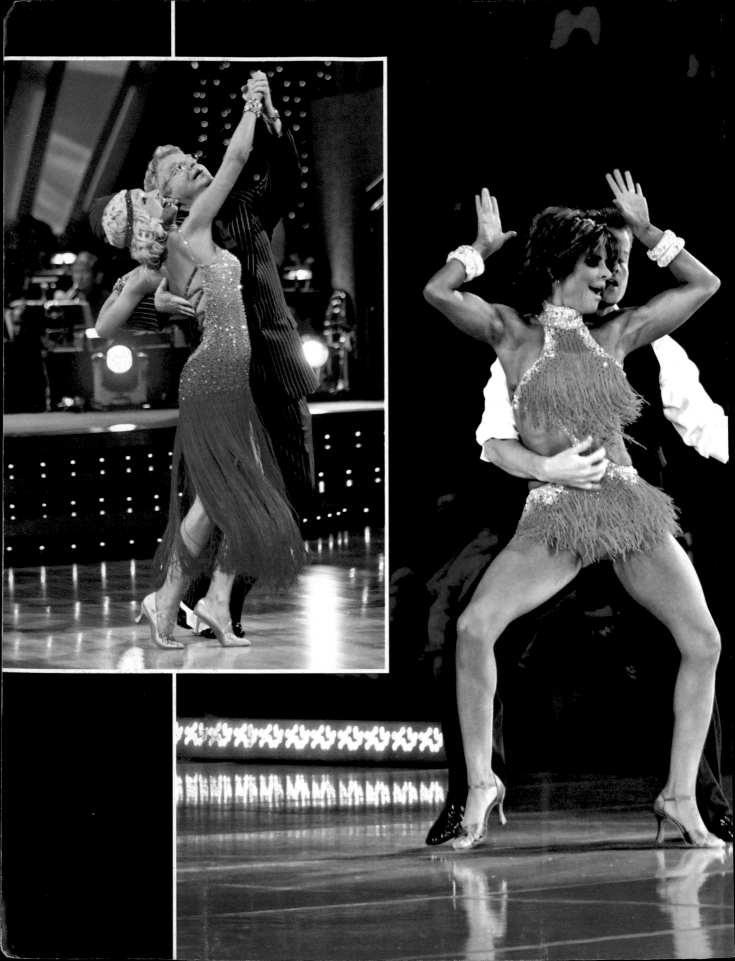

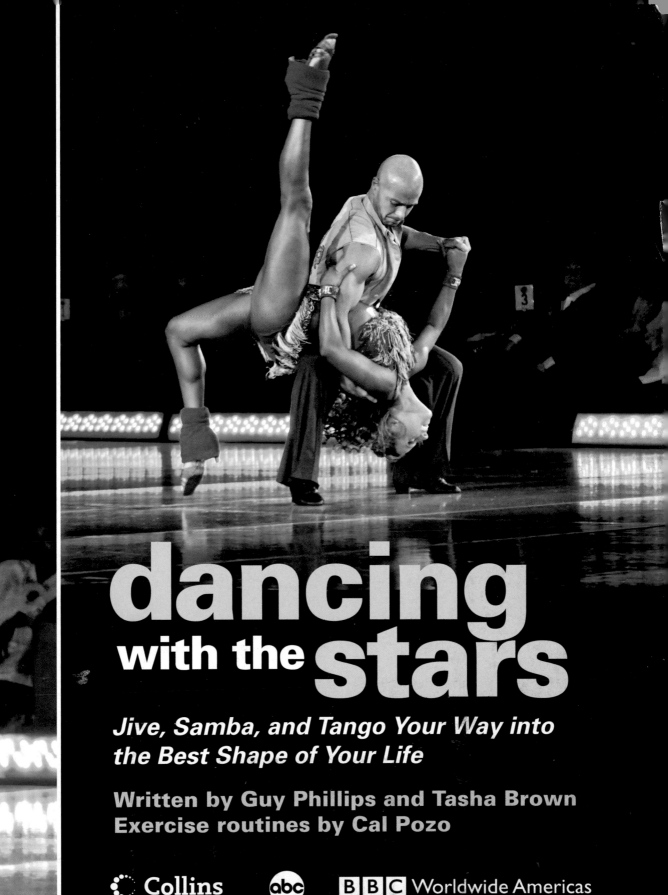

dancing
with the stars

Jive, Samba, and Tango Your Way into the Best Shape of Your Life

Written by Guy Phillips and Tasha Brown
Exercise routines by Cal Pozo

Collins
An Imprint of HarperCollins Publishers

abc

BBC Worldwide Americas

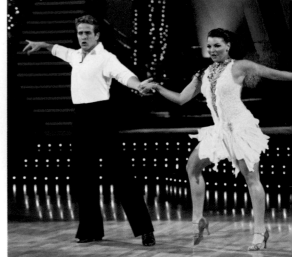

dancing with the stars

For information, address HarperCollins Publishers,
10 East 53rd Street, New York, NY 10022.

HarperCollins books may be purchased for educational,
business, or sales promotional use. For information please write:
Special Markets Department, HarperCollins Publishers,
10 East 53rd Street, New York, NY 10022.

FIRST EDITION

Designed by Richard J. Berenson, Berenson Design & Books, LLC and
The Stonesong Press, LLC

Library of Congress Cataloging-in-Publication Data

Dancing with the stars : jive, samba, and tango your way into the best
shape of your life.
       p. cm.
ISBN 978-0-06-143525-6
1. Ballroom dancing. 2. Dance--Latin America. 3. Physical fitness.
4. Dancing with the stars (Television program) I. Title.

        GV1751.D28 2007
        793.3'3--dc22

                                            2007023445

07 08 09 10 11 ❖/QW   10 9 8 7 6 5 4 3 2 1

contents

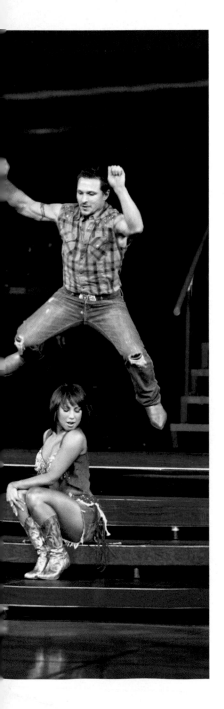

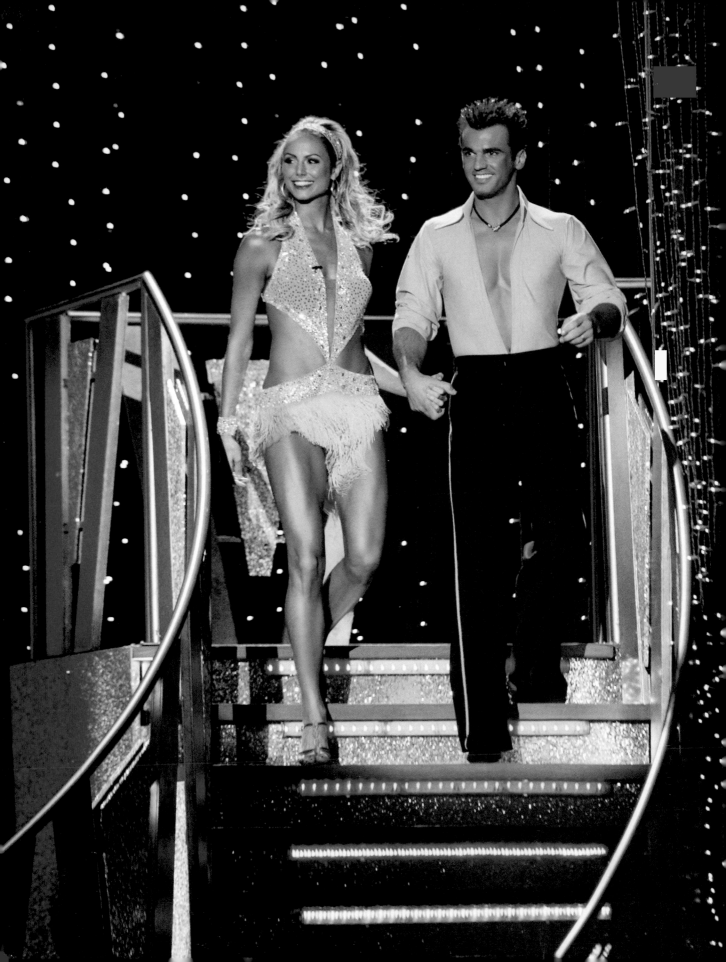

foreword

Dancing with the Stars has captivated audiences across the country with dazzling performances, timeless glamour, and its unique ability to enthrall the entire family. While the spotlights shine most brightly in the ballroom, the real drama is often played out in training, as the couples struggle to master this new art in which they have become immersed.

The cast is drawn from all walks of life, including sports stars, icons of the silver screen, singers, models, and journalists. From the young to the distinguished, they are a diverse group brought together by the great leveler of a common challenge. No matter who you are, there is someone on the show whose journey you can relate to, someone to identify with and be inspired by.

Dancing with the Stars has encouraged legions of fans to take up ballroom dancing themselves, whether to Waltz like Jerry, Jive like Lisa, or Quickstep like old "twinkle toes" Emmitt Smith. It is hard not to be amazed by the transformations many of the stars have gone through and the incredible physical condition of the professional dancers. During the course of the show, many pounds have been lost on the dance floor, as the hard work in training has paid dividends not only in better technique, but also in improved strength, flexibility, and stamina.

This book celebrates some of the greatest performances from the first four seasons and will help to make you a more knowledgeable judge yourself in seasons to come. If you are also inspired enough to take to the dance floor, or simply want to get a dancer's body yourself, we have included a classic dancers' workout that provides a fun, effective, and complete way to get ballroom-fit. You could also combine these workouts with your usual routine, or better still, with dance classes, to complete your own transformation.

So don't just sit there and watch the stars perform, get up and dance like one yourself!

We hope you continue to enjoy watching *Dancing with the Stars* on ABC and come to visit us when the tour comes to town . . . Live!

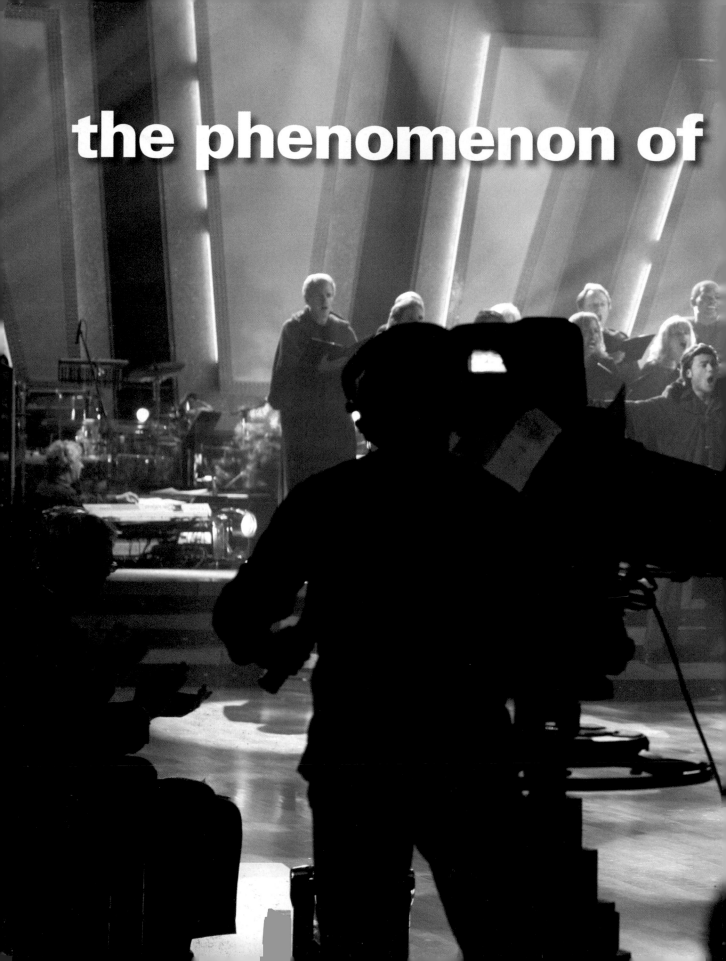

the phenomenon of

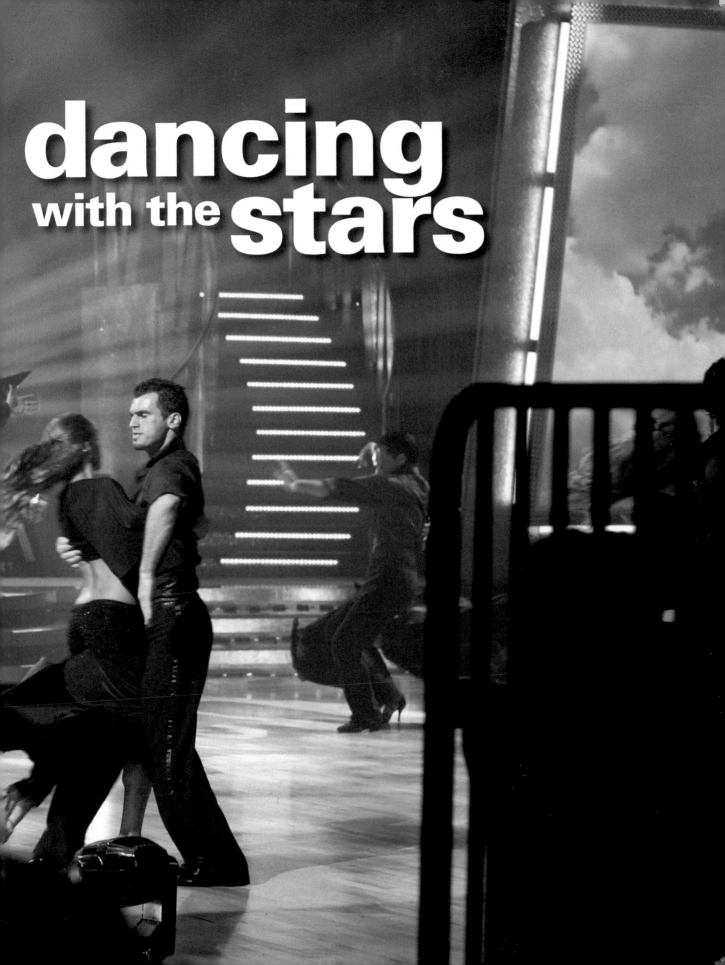

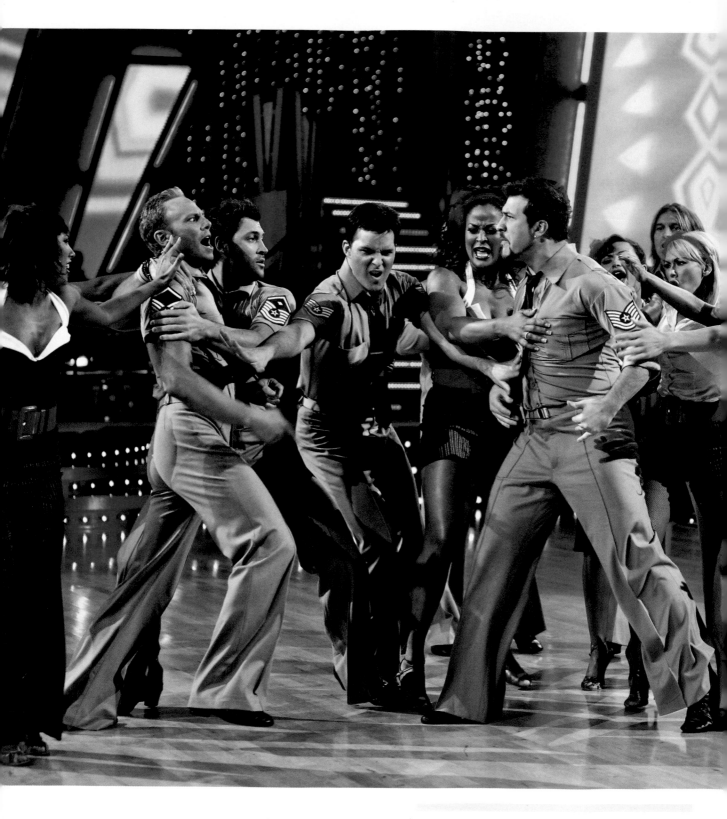

Ian and Joey stage a fight over Cheryl's affections in a nostalgic and fun group Swing.

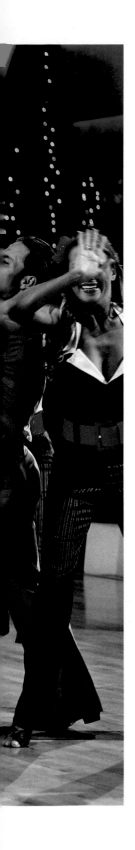

the history of the show

While brainstorming ideas in the fall of 2003, producers in the BBC entertainment department came up with the concept of bringing an old classic, *Come Dancing,* out from the vaults. *Come Dancing* was first shown on the BBC in 1949, and was primarily designed to educate the public about the joys of dancing. In 1953 the series introduced competition, in which winners were picked from the live national finals and became proud owners of the *Come Dancing* trophy. The show was one of the longest running in British television history, finally coming to an end in 1995, when it had begun to feel dated and audiences dwindled.

The BBC producers, led by Executive Producer Karen Smith, realized that the best way to update the show and grab the attention of viewers of all ages was to throw celebrities into the mix. So they devised the mega-hit *Strictly Come Dancing.*

By putting famous stars together with professional dancers, the new show was able to engage and entertain a far wider audience than simply dance fans. The traditional appeal of watching a dazzling dance performance was enhanced by witnessing the journeys of amateurs learning new skills. The fact that the amateurs were known for their success in other fields made the fish-out-of-water stories all the more compelling. One of the biggest additions was

"With dazzling costumes, fantastic performances, celebrity gossip, behind-the-scenes training, and contemporary music played by a live band, it can be a wonderful and inspirational escape from everyday reality for [people of] all ages."
Izzie Pick, co-executive producer

filming the backstage training so that viewers could really see the trials and tribulations of the stars learning their dances, the relationships that formed between the couples, and their wonderful transformation from the sweaty training to the glamorous live show.

coming to the usa

The huge success of *Strictly Come Dancing* made it the perfect candidate to follow other UK hits like *Who Wants to Be a Millionaire, The Weakest Link,* and *American Idol* over the Atlantic to be remade for American audiences. Several of the biggest hits of recent years had been created in the UK. However, the idea of ballroom dancing on US network prime time met with some skepticism when first pitched by the UK executive producer, Richard Hopkins.

"For a while, I considered the show, but just didn't believe a series about ballroom dancing would work in the US. But then I sat down with the executive producer and he convinced me that it was a 'leap of faith.' I'll never forget that. He asked me to just sit down and watch an entire episode. The next day, I had the whole department watch a full episode and we fell in love with it. We turned to each other and said, 'Are we crazy?' And we all loved it so much that we decided to take a risk and try it."

—Andrea Wong, executive vice president, Alternative Programming, Specials and Late Night, ABC Entertainment

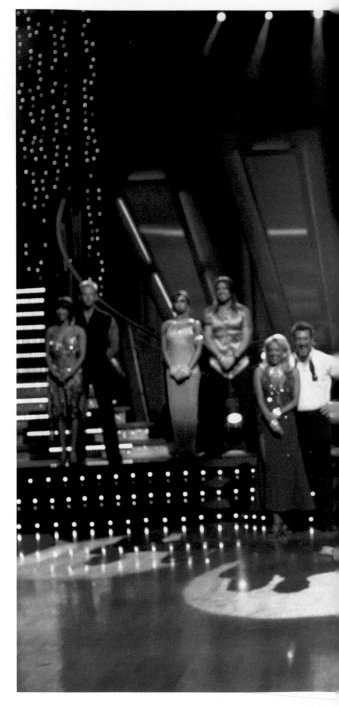

Hosts Tom Bergeron and Samantha Harris.

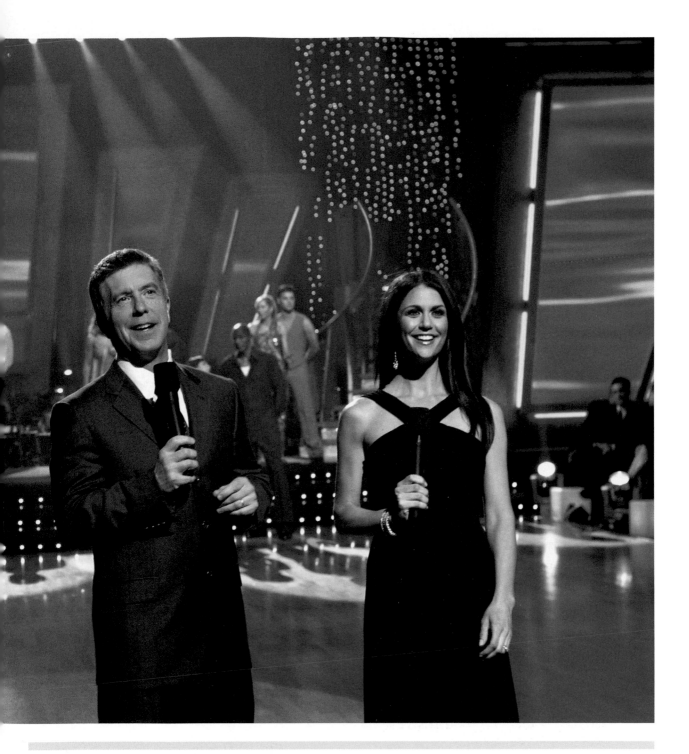

"*Although a long-time fitness enthusiast and lover of cardio classes at the gym, I have long admired the toned definition of a dancer's body. Since watching the pros on* Dancing with the Stars *up close, I have been awed by what incredible athletes they are. Witnessing the amazing physical transformations our celebs have made in tightening and sculpting their bodies after training for the show proves just how effective dance is to get in shape and be fit.*"
—Samantha Harris, Co-Host of *Dancing with the Stars* and three-time cover model for *Muscle & Fitness HERS Magazine*

The show had already been turned down three times by US networks, but the stars aligned at ABC, where executives saw its uniqueness as a strength. John Saade at ABC summed up best just how different the show would be: "Like an alien space-craft has landed at nine p.m. on a Wednesday night."

The ABC team wanted to maintain the uniquely British feel and asked for little to be changed from the UK show. The set, complete with audience members sitting at candlelit tables in cocktail attire, the catchy theme song, and the comforting choice of host were all a must. So it seemed only natural to bring over a team of top British producers. Conrad Green joined Richard Hopkins as executive producer, and Izzie Pick came directly from the UK series to produce, along with senior video producer Rob Wade, studio producer Matilda Zoltowski, field producer Jo Sungkur, and director Alex Rudzinski.

The executive producers Conrad and Izzie are very superstitious and carry a lucky stone and a lucky bag to every live show for luck.

By March 2005 the fifteen-thousand-square-foot stage 46 at CBS studios in Hollywood, California, was booked (right next door to the *American Idol* studio), and the production crew had been hired. Tom Bergeron and Lisa Cannin were selected to host, and completing the picture were the six celebrities who had been brave enough to take a leap of faith with this strange British import, and see in it the same potential that ABC had. They were boy-bander Joey McIntyre, soap star Kelly Monaco, model Rachel Hunter, reality-star Trista Rehn Sutter, boxer Evander Holyfield, and *Seinfeld*'s John O'Hurley.

It was an eclectic mix, but one that the producers thought would cover the wide range of audience appeal.

The stars on Season one had no idea what to expect on the first show day, but Joey McIntyre was brave enough to be the first on the floor.

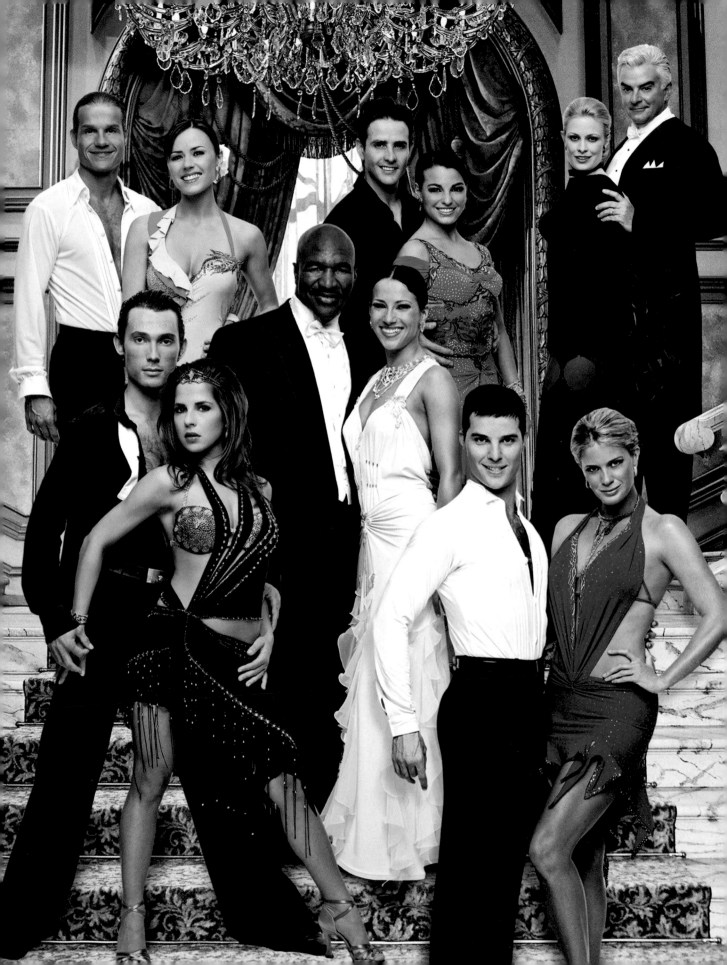

One of the keys to making the show work was the voting system. In the UK, the producers had wanted to avoid the show being purely a popularity contest and had worked hard to find a way of balancing the dancing performance with the popularity of the stars taking part. Traditionally, in ballroom dancing competitions, the competitors are scored based on their dancing ability, so the creative decision was reached to give fifty percent of the vote to the viewers and the other fifty percent to the judges. This unique scoring system allowed the viewers to vote with their hearts based on personality and performance, while the judges could concentrate on technique and dance ability. That meant anyone could take part in the show, great dancer or not.

Also unique to *Dancing with the Stars* is that each individual dance style has its own specific requirements and basic steps that only the judges are qualified to watch for. There are ten different ballroom and Latin-American dances, and the producers wanted each one to be as true to its original roots as possible to avoid them all merging into one wild Freestyle. The judges' input limits the couples' showboating and ensures they are challenged each week to learn the different steps and moves required. Although Joey Fatone's butt sticking out might have worked against him in the ballroom dances, he shone in his Latin-American Samba. The guidelines also mean that the performances have real depth and variety each week.

> Len and Bruno had to fly back to the UK eight times during season three to judge the UK series—a total of 128,000 miles. That's the equivalent of flying around the world five times for each of them!

Two judges from the UK show, Len Goodman and Bruno Tonioli, were also brought to the US and teamed up with Carrie Ann Inaba to complete the panel.

Dancing with the Stars premiered on ABC on June 1, 2005, to an audience of over thirteen million, making it the most successful summer debut ever for a reality series. The audience continued to grow throughout the competition and it finished its run at number one in the ratings.

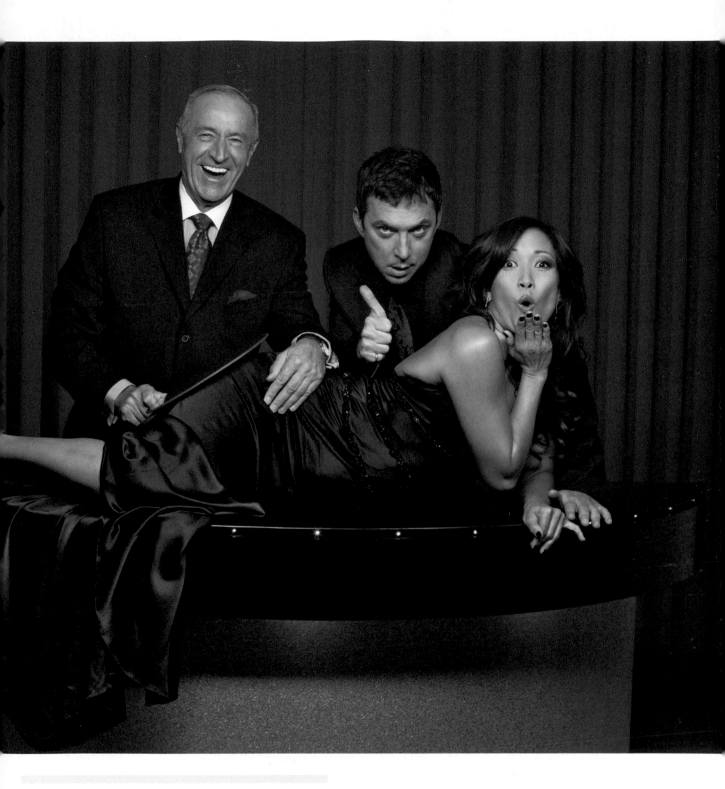

Judge Bruno Tonioli (center), flanked by Head Judge
Len Goodman (left) and Judge Carrie Ann Inaba (right).

behind the ballroom

The couple twirling their way around the dance floor are only the tip of the iceberg on a show with 2 hosts, 3 judges, a 15-piece orchestra, up to 22 dancers, a production crew of over 200, and a studio audience of 550. The logistics involved to bring all these people and their equipment together for a live show are immense.

The journey to the ballroom begins with finding the right stars to take to the floor, a challenge for talent producers Conrad Green, Izzie Pick, and talent producer Deena Katz.

"Casting Dancing with the Stars *is part planning, part inspiration, and part luck. We never know how good our stars will actually be at dancing before they appear on the show, so we can only go on conversations we have had with them, and their willingness to take part. It is hard to predict who will want to take part—we never expected Jerry Rice, Tatum O'Neal, or Jerry Springer to see it as something they may want to do, but you find passion for dance in the most surprising places!*

We are approached by lots of people, but at first we look for a few stars that embody how we would want the cast to look, and then we aim to cast around them. We also target a few people who are surprising, or we wouldn't necessarily expect to do the show. With these 'Hail Marys' we don't expect much return, but if they come off we use these as tent-poles of the cast and build the rest of the stars around them. By definition they are people you don't expect to want to take part and are essential for getting people excited about the early shows. Jerry Springer came about like this—we didn't have a clue that he was worried about preparing a dance for his daughter's wedding, but that was what spurred him to consider our offer from

The final performance is the tip of the iceberg, as the couples train relentlessly to perfect their steps.

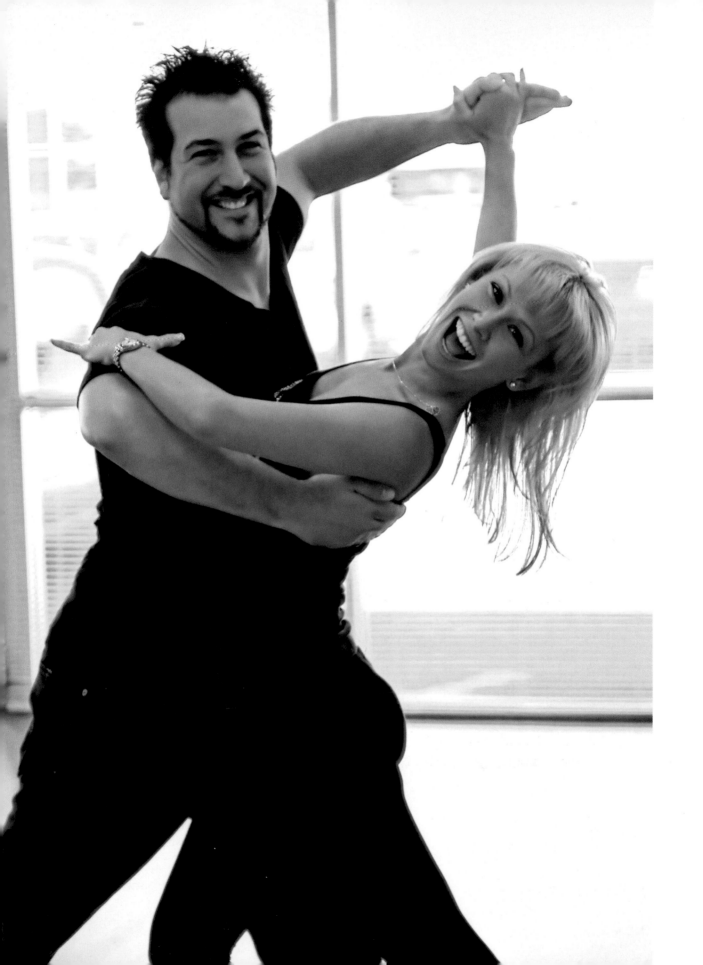

the many that come his way. We read a false story in a British tabloid that we had booked Heather Mills to appear on the show, but that got us thinking that she would be a great story, and really inspiring to watch. Our theme for season four was to make the cast as diverse as possible so we put out an offer and were astonished when she said yes . . . Sometimes the tail does wag the dog!

Dancing with the Stars *has a really wide audience, and one of the show's strengths is that we can cast people from all corners of the entertainment world and, to some extent, bring their fans to our show. We always look at sports stars, as their athleticism and competitive instincts give the show a real edge. Musicians are great as well, as they're usually decent dancers and understand performance. Actors are very strong competitors due to their appeal and their performance abilities, and we try to book across all ages to appeal to the widest possible range of our audience. When we have a few bookings in place, we then work on trying to balance the cast by age, look, and expected ability. Fate takes a big hand in the casting— Master P became involved when his son was unable to do the show, and John Ratzenberger was able to step in for Vincent Pastore after a previous commitment went away. We always try to meet with stars before they commit to the project as it's really important for them to understand the huge amount of work that the show entails behind the scenes. At this stage we ask them whether they have had formal ballroom or Latin dance training. Often entertainers have had some dance training in their careers but only if they have had extensive training in the dances we use on the show would we consider it unfair for them to enter the competition.*

We've given up trying to predict who will win the show, as I've always been hopelessly wrong. I think that's the charm of the series—anybody can cross the finish line first, and success depends on a peculiar mixture of dance talent, popularity, and the ability to pace yourself well on the show.

—Conrad Green, Executive Producer, talking about casting the show

Paula Abdul often comes backstage to watch the show during breaks in *American Idol,* **which is filmed in the studio next door.**

Jerry came on the show so he could learn to dance well enough to waltz with his daughter Katie on her wedding day, but this Samba shows how much Kym widened his repertoire along the way.

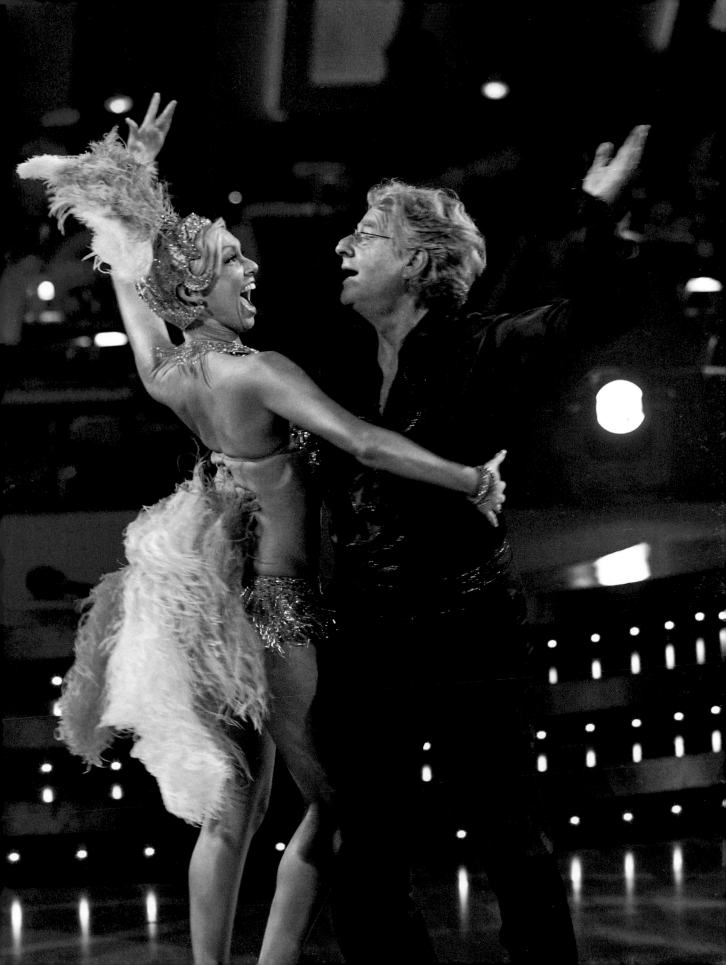

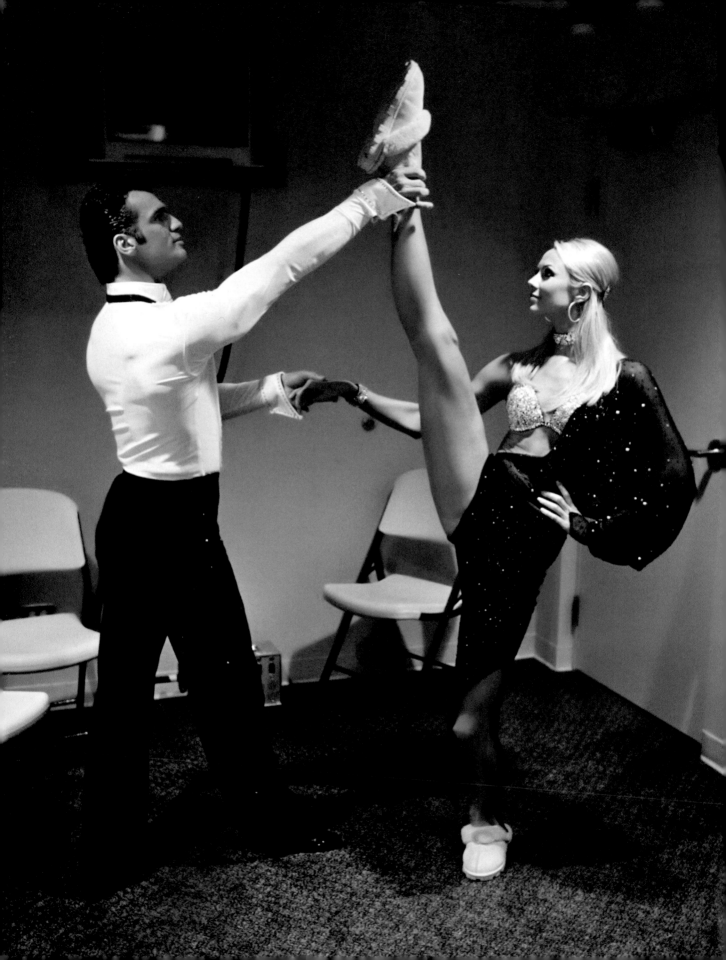

On a live network show of this complexity there is no room for error, and so preparations are exhaustive. Show days start with full dress rehearsals, where the script, running order, music, and dancing are perfected. Ten cameras follow the action in the ballroom, and rehearsals ensure that everyone is in the correct place and on time without tripping over or filming one another. Camera operators are choreographed into the action as tightly as the performers, with cameras often stepping out onto the floor with the stars, or ducking out of shot behind the audience members. Try to spot the cameras next time you watch the show!

On season two, all of the camera operators got locked out of the studio minutes before the show and had to persuade the security guards to let them back in.

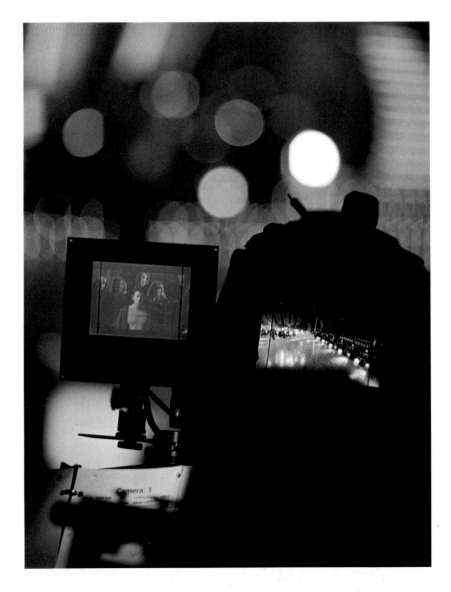

Tony Dovolani and Stacy Keibler warm up backstage. Stacy did swap the slippers for dance shoes before hitting the ballroom.

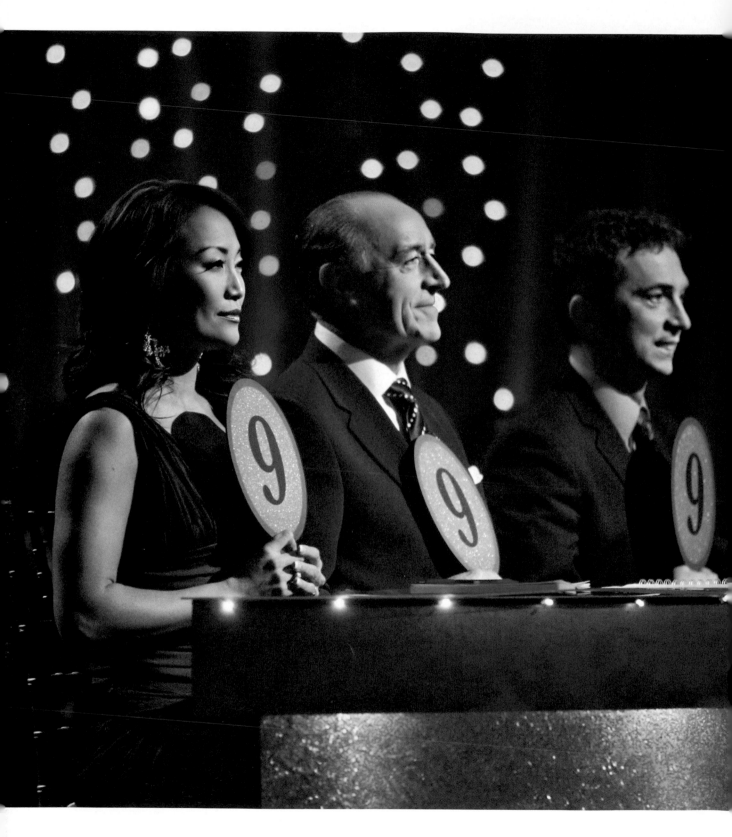

the judges' scores

The way the judges score performances is a highly complicated and technical process. The second the couples complete their routine, each judge types their score into a keypad on their desk. That score is then verified by an independent adjudicator through a computer system behind the audience seating. The adjudicator adds the three scores together and verifies the total before relaying it to the producers in the live control room, who also verify with the ABC broadcast standards representative. The score is then keyed into the graphics machine and relayed to Samantha Harris in the backstage area. The whole process takes less than a minute. The correct score is always the score keyed into the computer by the judges.

On season two, after Tia and Maks danced, Carrie Ann Inaba keyed in her score as usual, but when it came time for her to hold up her paddle, she forgot the score she had given and held up the wrong paddle. This meant that the score seen on screen didn't match the paddle she was holding. The next day on the results show, Carrie Ann held up a "Sorry" paddle! Just goes to prove that the judges are human too.

Poor Maks was on the receiving end of another scoring malfunction on season four, too. After Laila and Maks' Cha-cha, the scoring process took place as usual. But after interviewing them, Samantha Harris, who had received the score earlier, forgot that the scores had not been revealed to the viewers, and let the cat out of the bag in her excitement. Luckily, Samantha quickly realized what she had said, and explained all to the viewers.

Judge Carrie Ann Inaba, Head Judge Len Goodman, and Judge Bruno Tonioli show their approval.

The training teams follow every step of the stars' journeys, filming each training session in order to create the video segments that introduce each couple's live dance performance and tell their stories. Working in shifts to cover every couple 24-7, the training teams witness the highs and lows, and are responsible for showing the audience how the couples are getting on. If you are looking for gossip, these are the people to speak to!

Training teams are the producers who go out in the field and film all the stars' training. Shadowing them throughout their journey, the teams are on hand to document the highs and lows and to show the audience the stars' individual personalities.

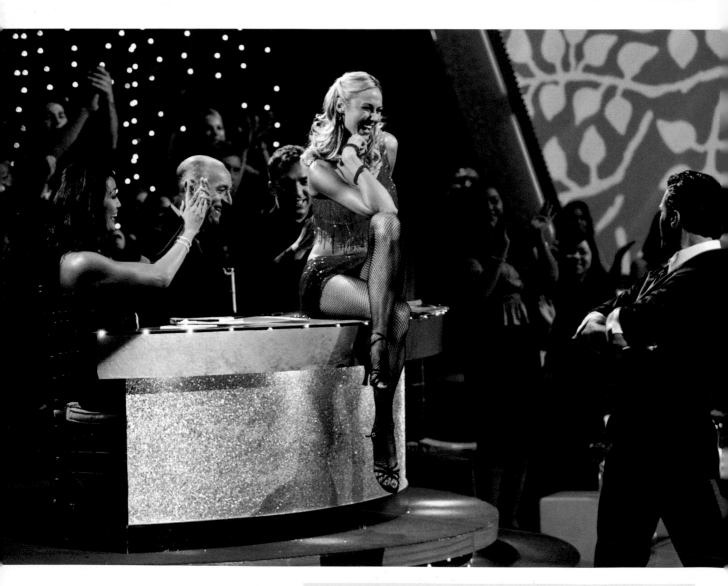

Stacy Keibler makes sure she has the Judges' full attention.

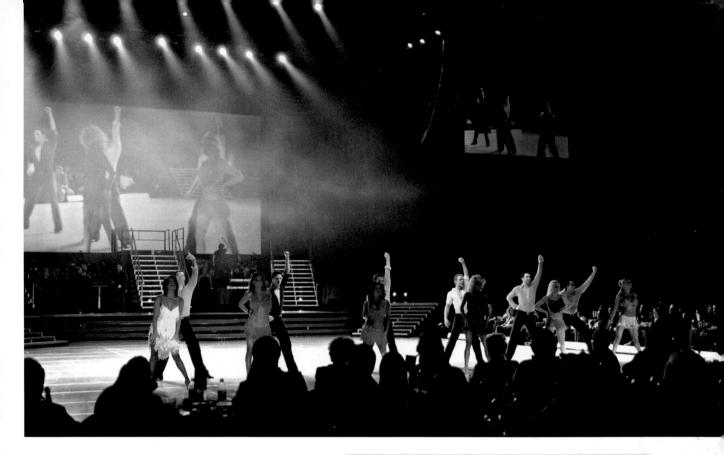

the music

The music is a huge element in creating the magic in the ballroom, and the use of contemporary songs to complement the classic dance tunes is unique in the dance world. Months before each season, the producers submit a list of hundreds of songs to the music editor, who identifies the tempo and style of each song to see if it can be matched to any of the ballroom dances. The stars and dancers are then asked for a list of their favorites, which are accommodated whenever possible. The final track choices are edited down to a one-minute-and-thirty-second version, the tempo is corrected to match the dance style, and then the song is scored by the Tony Award–winning musical director Harold Wheeler.

> The first time the stars ever hear the band's version of their song is on the actual day of the show.

The music request process from the celebrities and professionals is often a highly contentious issue. Some songs are very popular with all the couples on any given week, while others are rejected by all of them. The producers often spend many hours bartering and making deals with the couples over what tracks they can have each week. Sometimes the competitors need to be persuaded to try unusual tracks, which often turn out to be the most successful performances. Who'd have thought you could Tango to the theme of *Star Wars,* or that "Lust for Life" would provide the perfect accompaniment to Harry Hamlin's Quickstep?

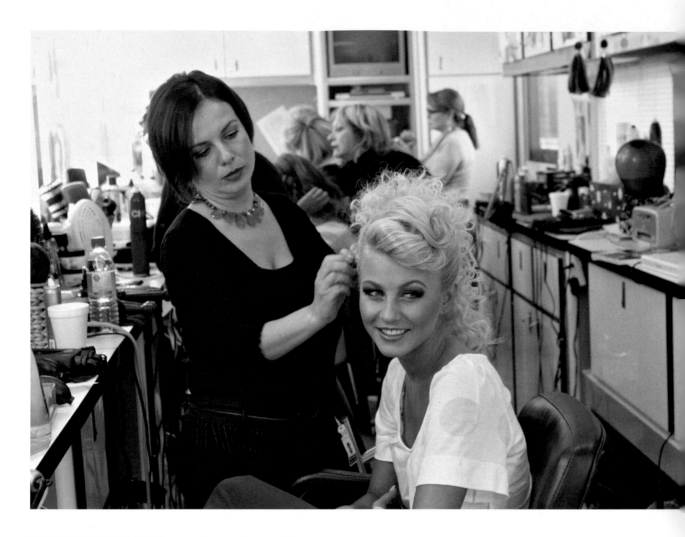

Julianne Hough, the winner of Season four, gets the finishing touches on her hair.

the look

Costumes, hair, and makeup play an important role in creating the *Dancing with the Stars* look, and artists in each department work closely together to achieve that look. It is distinct from the world of competition dancing, and it reflects the mix of contemporary and classic music. The makeup and hair have been updated to reflect modern Hollywood trends, and many looks take inspiration from the 1920s and 30s, blending periods to create a stunning retro style. The bodies are all darkly tanned and multilayered in tone because of the hard stage lights and to emphasize the physical movements, and the hairstyles are styled and pinned as though the dancers were doing stunts. Head of the makeup department, Melanie Mills, and head of the hair department, Mary Guerrero, describe the look best with their motto, "Hollywoodize and Glamorize."

Maksim Chmerkovskiy lends a hand with the makeup brush.

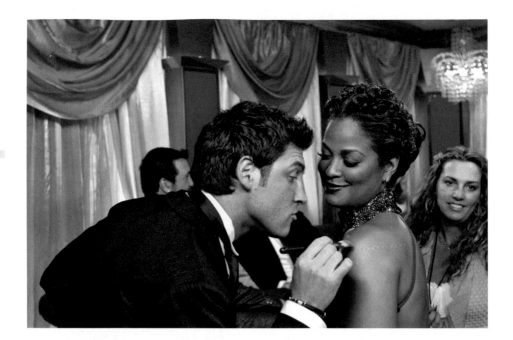

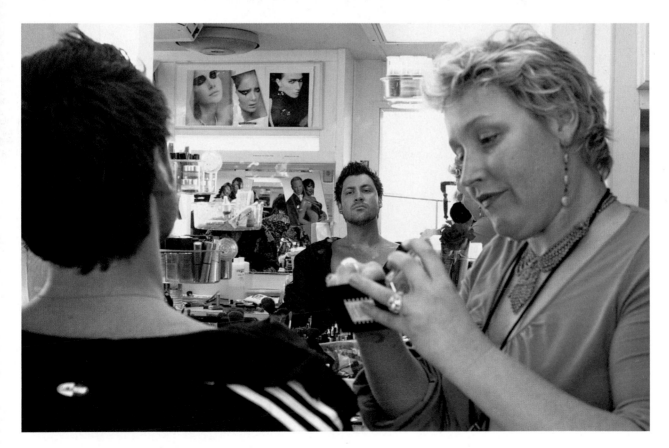

Maksim getting ready to perform with the help of Melanie Mills, Head of the makeup department.

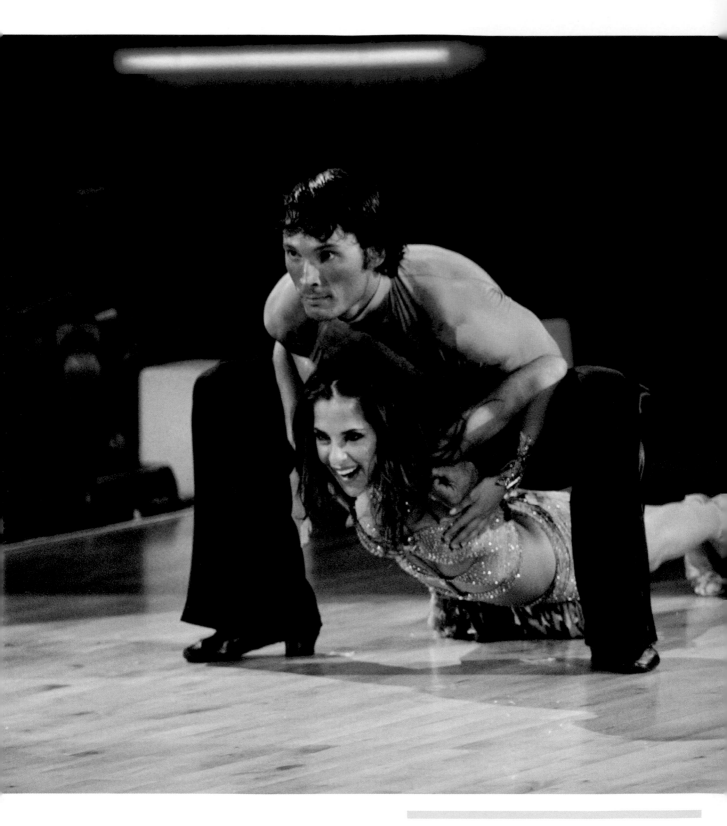

Kelly Monaco cleverly adapts her choreography mid-performance to cover a wardrobe malfunction.

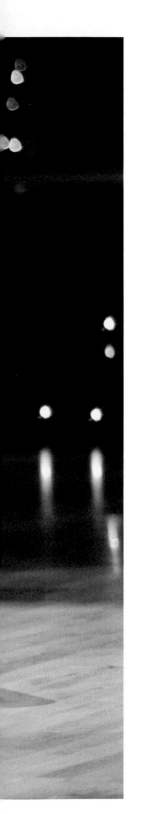

Costumes provide their own challenge, and each is created especially for the individual performance. All the women's and men's costumes are one-of-a-kind, custom-built garments. Each of the women's costumes has anywhere from one thousand to fifteen thousand rhinestones each, and some are made from silk and other delicate fabrics. Head designer Randall Christensen faces the daunting task of creating many unique new costumes each week that will be capable of withstanding the extreme physical demands of dancing. "Wardrobe malfunctions" are rare, and lessons have been learned from Kelly Monaco nearly losing her top in Season one.

To avoid any disasters should there be a wardrobe malfunction, the women always wear flesh covered "petals" on any body parts not deemed fit for public view.

The costumes need to have a great deal of give in them to allow flexibility, but not too much give, so all the men's pants are reinforced three times! Dresses can cost up to seven thousand dollars each, some with up to 130,000 Swarovski crystals glued on one at a time by hand—little wonder that they can take several days each to construct and fit. The tight schedule each week can lead to some last-minute panics. When Edyta Sliwinska's hair kept getting caught in Evander Holyfield's shirt during rehearsal, the wardrobe team had only a couple of hours before the live show to cut off the buttons and find an alternative. The show must go on!

The stars themselves have a great deal of input in the designs. Most of the stars love the way they look on the show, but sometimes they do have to be encouraged to embrace the ballroom style.

"They're [the costumes] very risqué—you're showing off your body— but they're beautiful. [The designer] is really good at taking your body and designing something that will flatter you and make you look good."—Stacy Keibler, *Dancing with the Stars,* Season two

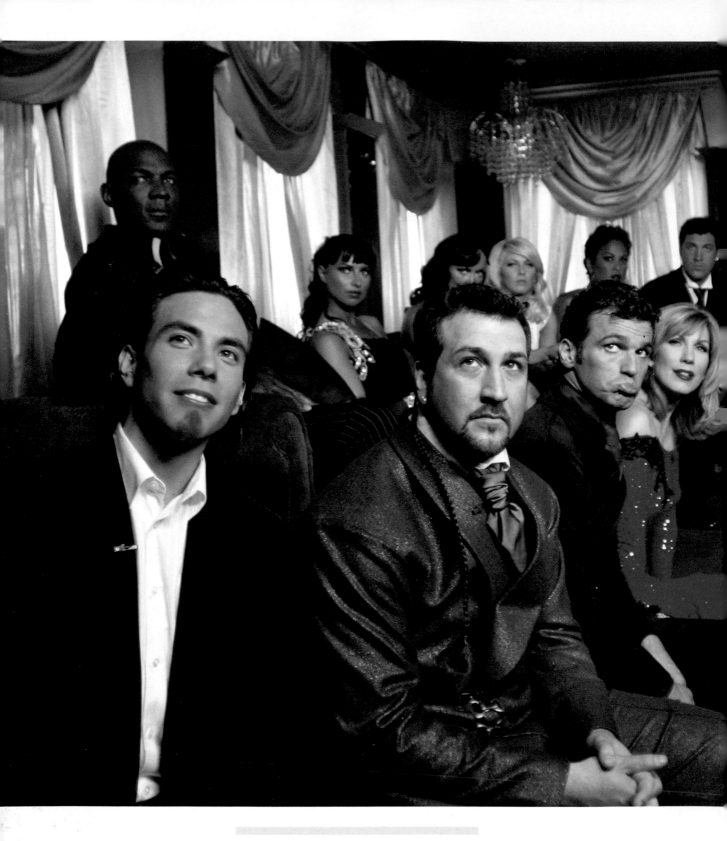

An anxious wait backstage for the scores.

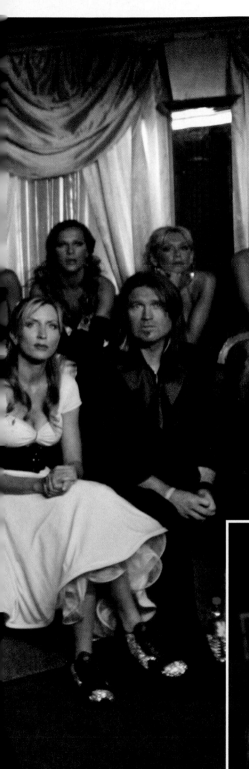

The dancing tour provided perhaps an even greater challenge for the show's costume supervisor, Kirstin Gallo, who hit the road to ensure all the delicate costumes were in perfect condition for performances night after night. Kirstin's first challenge was to build and tailor over three hundred costumes in the three weeks between the end of season three and the tour dress rehearsals. Every third show of the tour, each costume was hand washed and hand dried in a customized garment bag that was modified with a hair dryer to create a "dryer bag" so air could circulate around the costumes without shrinking or destroying them. In addition to the challenges of building and maintaining the costumes, there were over a hundred quick changes that took place in anywhere from under a minute to five minutes on the women's side alone.

George Hamilton had special pads built into his outfits to enhance the way his butt looked.

Edyta Sliwinska in the backstage makeup chair.

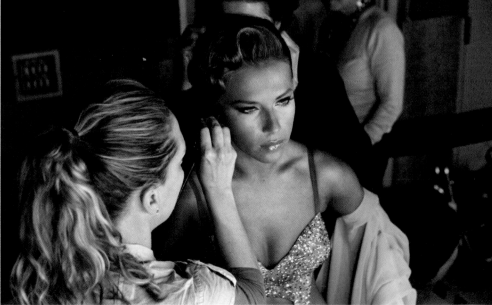

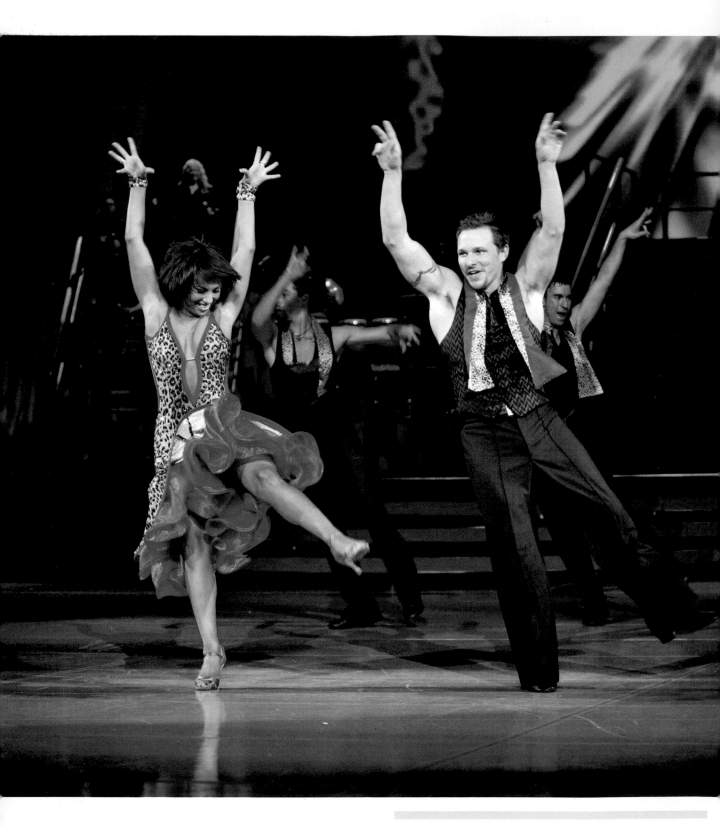

Winners of Season two, Drew Lachey and Cheryl Burke, have fun on the first Dancing with the Stars *Tour.*

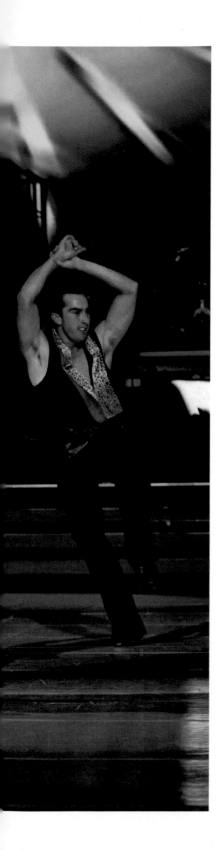

choreography

Each dance is choreographed by the professional dancers, who aim to showcase the strength of their star partners. With only four weeks to practice before each new season premieres, and five days to learn their new dances each week, the pressure to perform each night is intense.

The couples are given their dance style and music only the night of the results show, and dancers have only one night to create the choreography before they are back in the studio with their celebrity the next day. They must teach their celebrity and have the routine ready three days later for the director to look at and script. Halfway through the competition, they have to learn two dances in one week, so it's no wonder they're all exhausted.

Harry Hamlin had a dance floor installed in his garden so he could rehearse at night.

The most competitive stars manage to put in a huge amount of practice, with Emmitt Smith putting his NFL stamina to good use enduring 298 hours training, and Mario Lopez clocking in 347 hours during Season three. Blisters and sore muscles are an everyday problem, but all are part of the challenge. After such an exhausting and grueling regimen, it's little wonder that the stars leave the competition in such good shape.

"I came in carrying a couple extra pounds . . . but then as the weeks went on, that became a four-pack, a four-pack became a six, and a six became an eight. I think by the time that it was all said and done, I had, like, a twelve-pack."
—Drew Lachey, winner, *Dancing with the Stars*, Season two

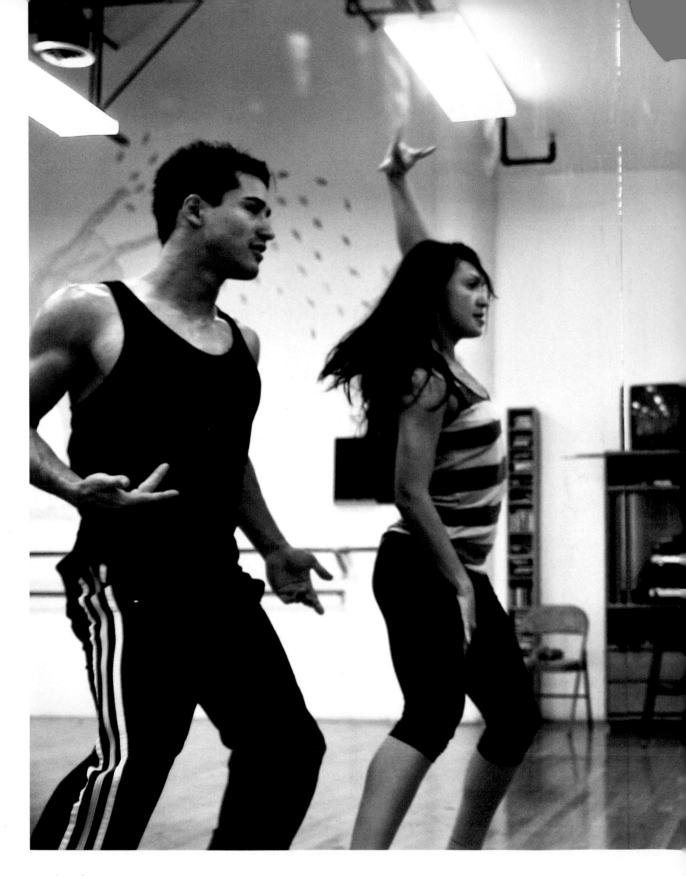

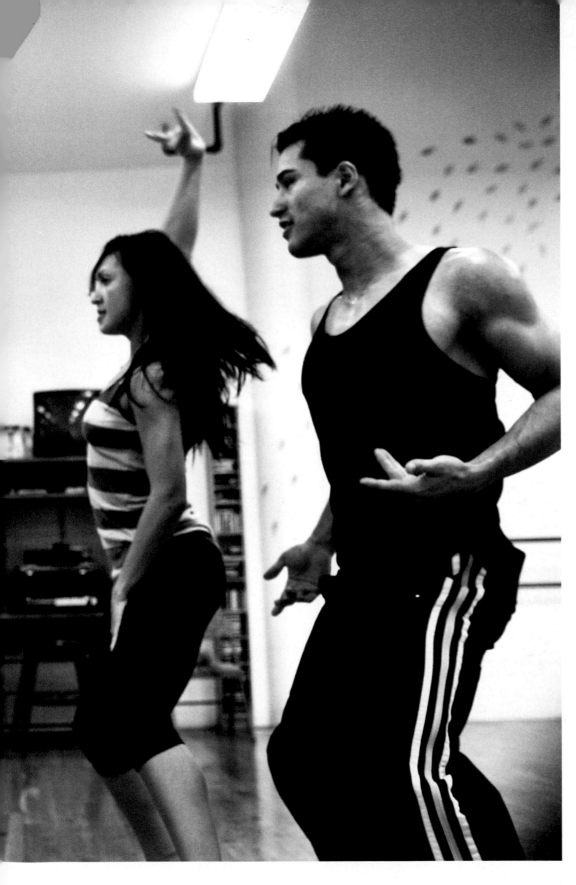

Mario Lopez and Karina Smirnoff made it look easy, but only after many hours of practice.

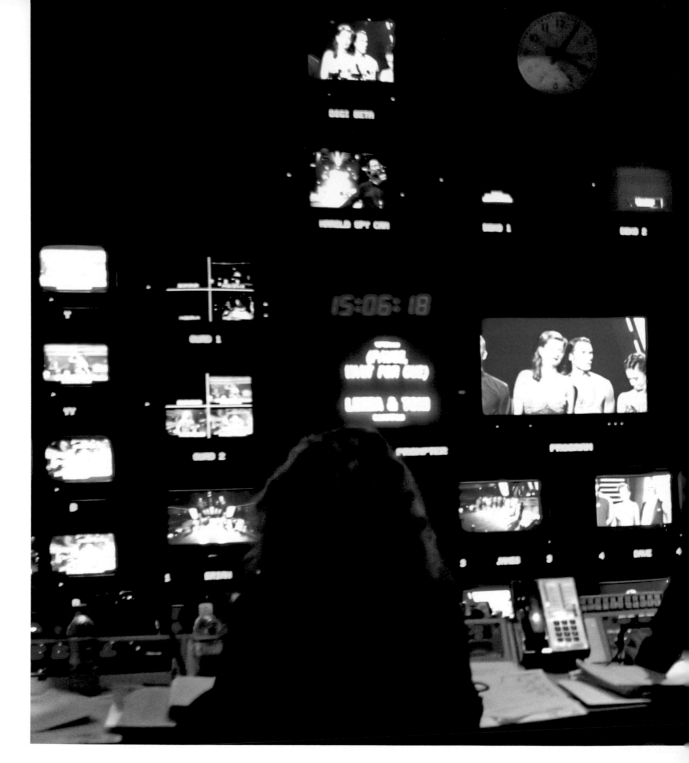

director's gallery

All the shows are live, the silence in the director's gallery in the minutes leading up to start time is a palpable sign of genuine tension. The silence is broken by the ten-second countdown, and for the remainder of the show, director Alex Rudzinski orchestrates an adrenaline-fueled team, constantly shout-

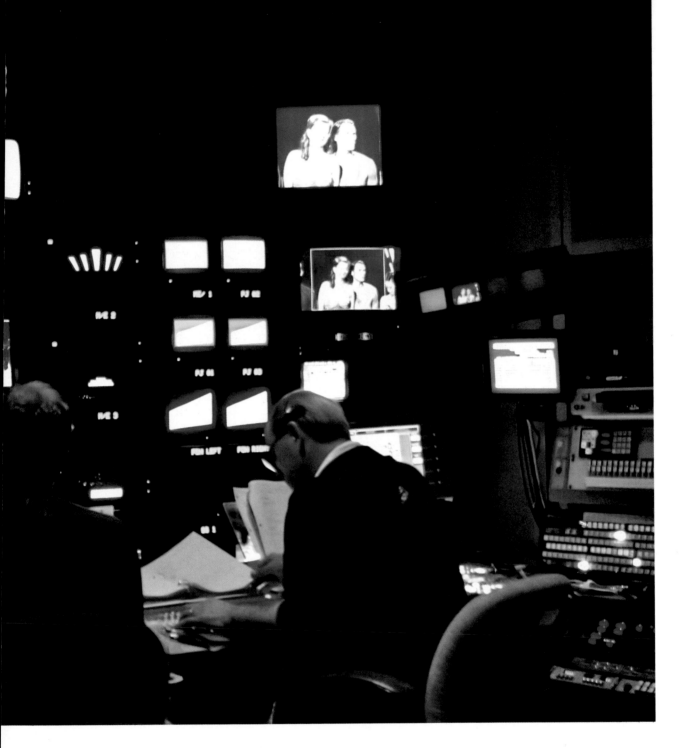

ing camera shots, speaking to the presenters, cuing the band, counting down to each training film, and making sure the runs go exactly as planned. Rudzinski makes up to 150 carefully planned camera cuts during each show to give the spectator the best possible view of the action.

Alex Rudzinski (center) calls the shots live in the gallery from the Director's chair.

life changes

"It's 'the guy that dances' now—people have forgotten about my football career. For the most part the topic of conversation for me is Dancing with the Stars."
—Emmitt Smith, NFL great and winner of Season three

Many of the stars have emerged from the show transformed, in fantastic physical shape, with a newfound confidence and passion in their lives. This confidence has led to many exciting opportunities for them.

Lisa Rinna auditioned for her dream role in the musical *Chicago* eight years ago, but couldn't keep up with the dancing required. Having learned to dance with Louis van Amstel on the series and performed on the *Dancing* tour, she was more than ready, and landed the role she so coveted on Broadway.

"Your sexual energy is better too, way better . . . people probably don't talk about that, but it's true. It needs to be mentioned. It's good for your sex life."
—Lisa Rinna, *Dancing with the Stars*, Season two and tour

Emmitt Smith and Cheryl Burke celebrate their win.

When Stacy Keibler was approached to compete on *Dancing with the Stars*, she was attempting to make the move from the world of the WWE (World Wrestling Entertainment) to the world of acting. She wanted to be taken seriously as an actress, so she wasn't sure that she wanted to do a reality show. Nevertheless, she took the plunge and hasn't looked back since.

"Dancing with the Stars *has changed my life in so many ways. I was able to let myself go. I've learned more about myself. I realized how hard I'm willing to work for something. And as for my career, I'm now able to do what I've always wanted to do."
—Stacy Keibler, *Dancing with the Stars*, Season two

After the show ended, Stacy's acting career took off. She was a regular on ABC's *What About Brian*, and continues to work in movies.

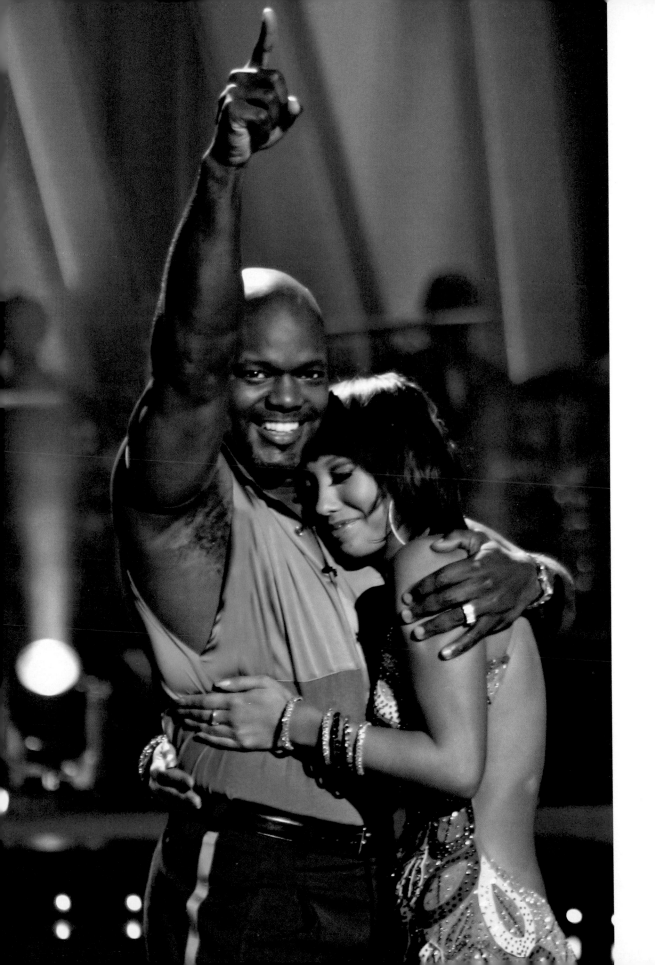

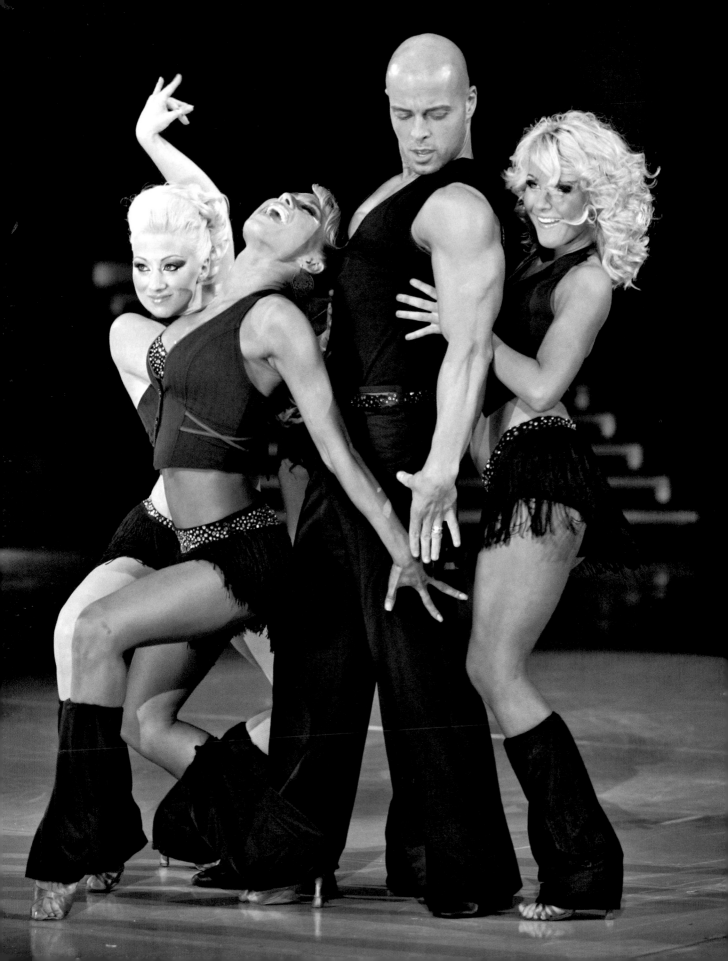

the beat goes on

Season two was even bigger than Season one, finishing as one of the top-ten most watched shows during the 2005–2006 season, and television's number one unscripted series of the season. The show's popularity continued to climb during season three, when it became the second-most watched program on television.

Dancing celebrated in December 2006 by going on a thirty-eight city live-arena tour across the US. Playing to sellout crowds, the tour brought more than three hundred thousand fans out to watch their favorite stars and dancers perform. The tour was choreographed by Louis van Amstel, a part of the TV show from the beginning and also a competitor in the original *Come Dancing*. Van Amstel was able to combine some old crowd favorites from the show, like Drew and Cheryl's "Save a Horse, Ride a Cowboy,"

> *"Ten thousand people a night just screaming and going nuts, loving it, a standing ovation every night . . . It's almost like going back to the boy-band days . . . except for a few less undergarments thrown on stage!"*
>
> —Drew Lachey, on the crowds' reactions

with spectacular, floor-filling, professional-group dances. The *Dancing* fans received the tour with unbridled enthusiasm.

Louis van Amstel and Karina Smirnoff used to be professional partners.

Ballroom and Latin dancing in the US have seen a massive surge in popularity as a result of the show. Dancing schools nationwide have seen a huge increase in the number of new dancers since the show started, with fans of *Dancing with the Stars* flocking to emulate their favorite moves. Perhaps the biggest contribution the show has made to the world of dancing has been to inspire so many young couples to take part in bringing glamour back to the ballroom.

Joey Lawrence on the Dancing with the Stars *Tour must be thinking about his old catchphrase—Whoa!*

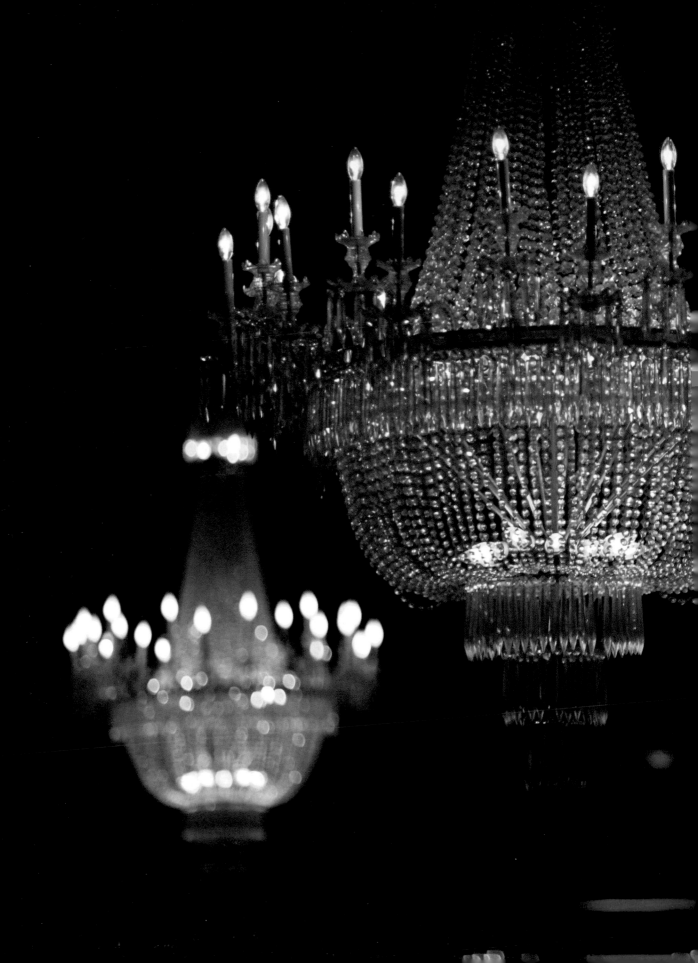

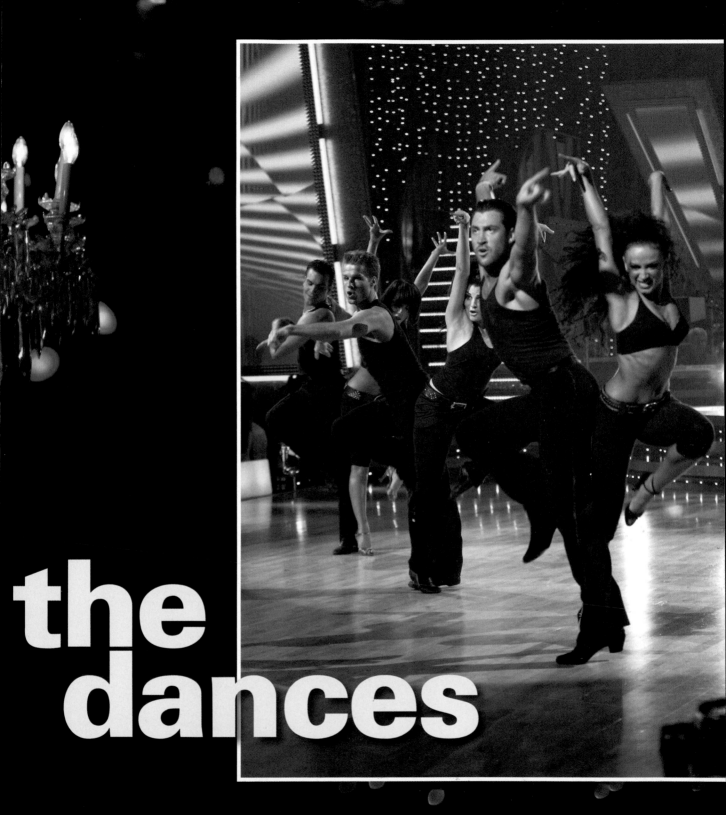

the
dances

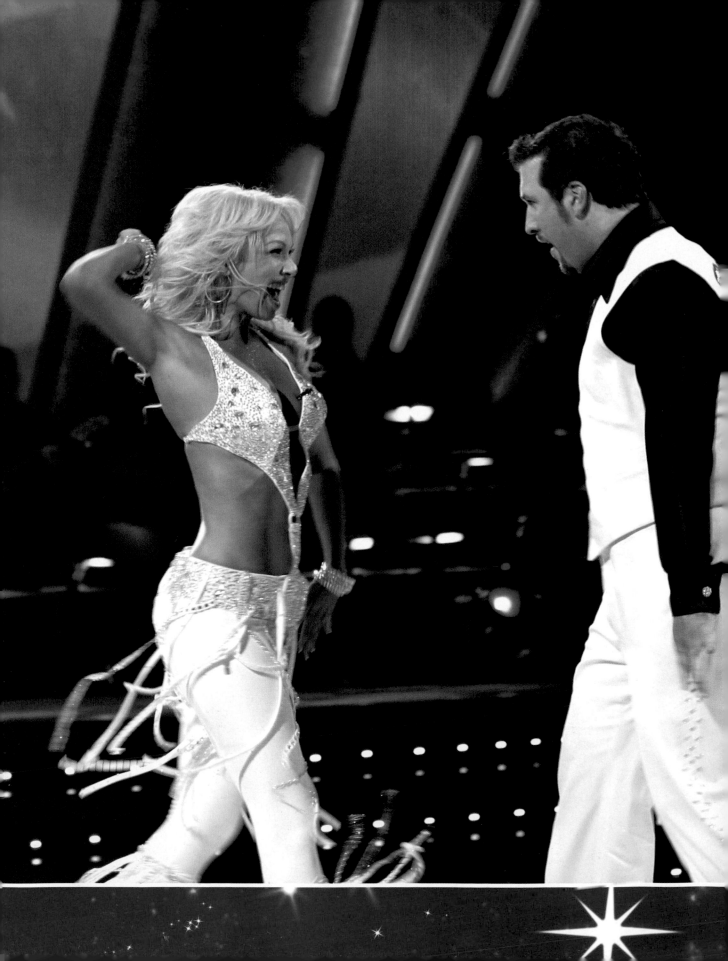

cha-cha

The Cha-cha is a number that allows the dancers to flirt and have fun.

Originally known as the Cha-Cha-Cha, the Cha-cha is an offshoot of the Mambo, and a cheeky cousin of the Rumba.

The dance became popular in the midfifties when a UK dance teacher, Pierre Lavelle, visited Cuba and discovered an easier Mambo danced with a triple step.

There are conflicting theories as to the derivation of the name. Some say it comes from a West Indian plant whose seedpods are called cha-cha and make a rattle that produces the cha-cha sound. Others believe it comes from the sound of sandals tapping on the floor.

Season 4 runner-up Joey Fatone set the standard early with professional partner Kym Johnson.

cha-cha

a cool cha-cha
Joey Fatone and Kym Johnson (Season 4, show 1)

It is always impressive when a star can come out in the first show and perform from the moment his feet hit the dance floor. Joey managed this rare feat with an energetic and stylish Cha-cha. Using all the experience he gained performing on tour with 'N Sync, Joey was able to forget the pressure and the fact that his microphone pack came loose halfway through the routine, and put in a debut strong enough to have the judges in raptures.

Scores of 8, 8, 8 put Joey and Kym at the top of the competition. A perfect start!

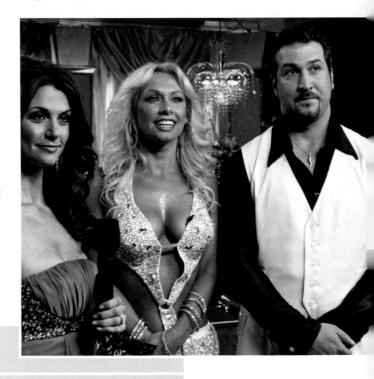

The tense wait was well worth it, as the Judges awarded scores of 8,8,8.

Judges' Comments

Carrie Ann Inaba: *"I think the competition just began right now, with you! It was charismatic, fun, energetic. I love your sense of humor."*

Len Goodman: *"The path to glory starts right here, and you've just taken an enormous step forward."*

Bruno Tonioli: *"This is really what it's all about. It's about performing; it's about selling; it's about being on it with the music and with your partner."*

Joey and Kym wore custom-made matching track suits in rehearsal to "intimidate" the competition.

A dramatic finish brought the crowd to their feet.

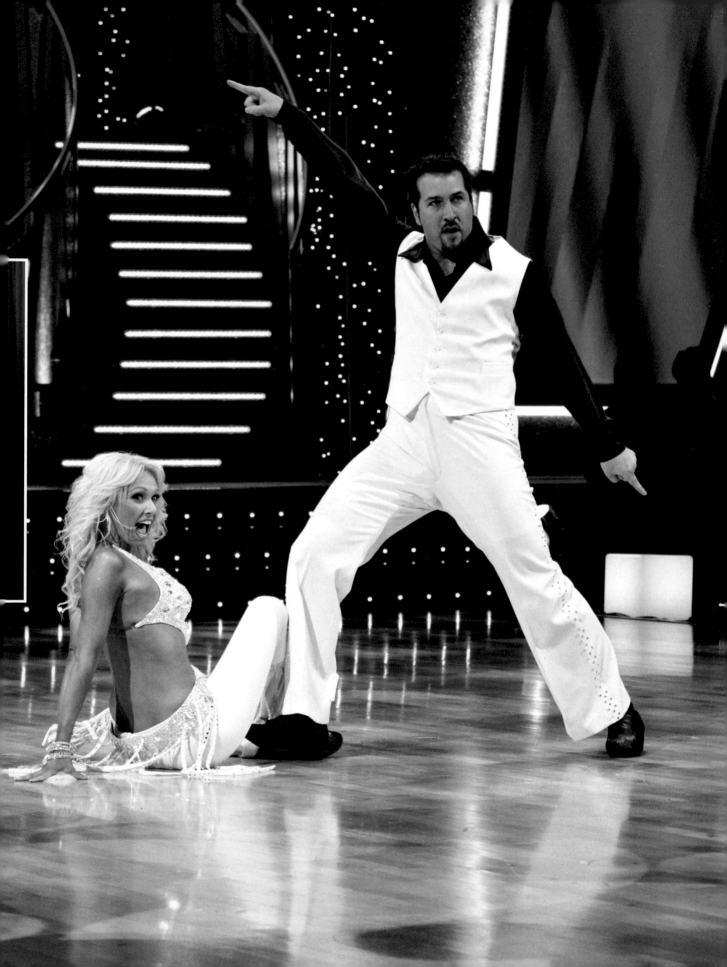

cha-cha
the look

Joey Fatone had a margarita machine in his trailer and made margaritas for the cast before the Results Show.

Kym and Joey's throwback to the seventies disco era was fun to design. Joey was open to doing whatever the costume designer wanted, including adding the rhinestone trim to his pants and a big "Fatone" to the back of his vest. He was having fun with the costumes from the very first episode. Kym's halter-neck jumpsuit with the big blinged-out belt was a tribute to the Abba era. It was a challenge to find the perfect trim for that piece.

Kym's hair was a very seventies Farrah Fawcett do—blow-dried, soft, upward curls. Her makeup was flirty and shimmering with a white iridescent and nude lip.

Cheryl Burke and Ian Ziering had a fantastic look for the Cha-cha in the fourth season. Cheryl had not worn black since her first season, and adding "nuts and bolts" to her costume was lots of fun. Because they were dancing to "Mony Mony," the look called for a bit more "rocker" and less ballroom. Ian wore basic black accented with a pyramid nailhead-studded belt. The chrome nailheads, stones, and pony beads were added on the fringed strips of fabric on Cheryl's costume to tie in with Ian's belt.

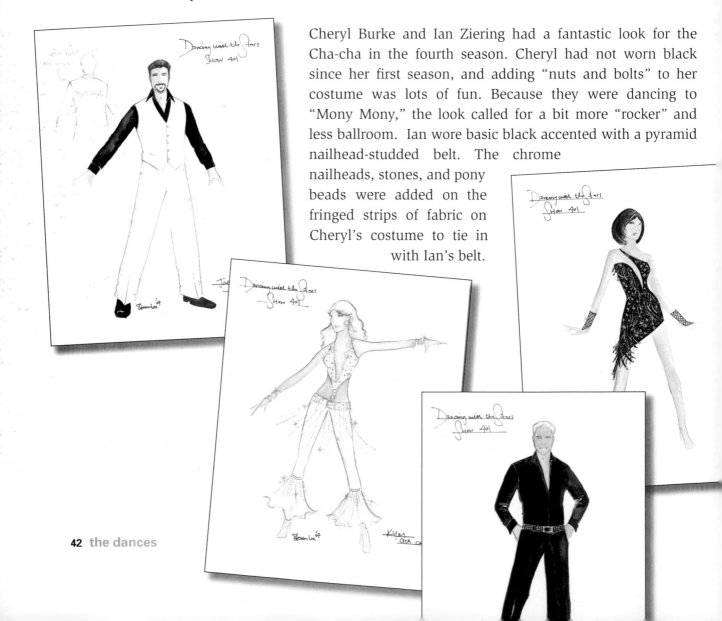

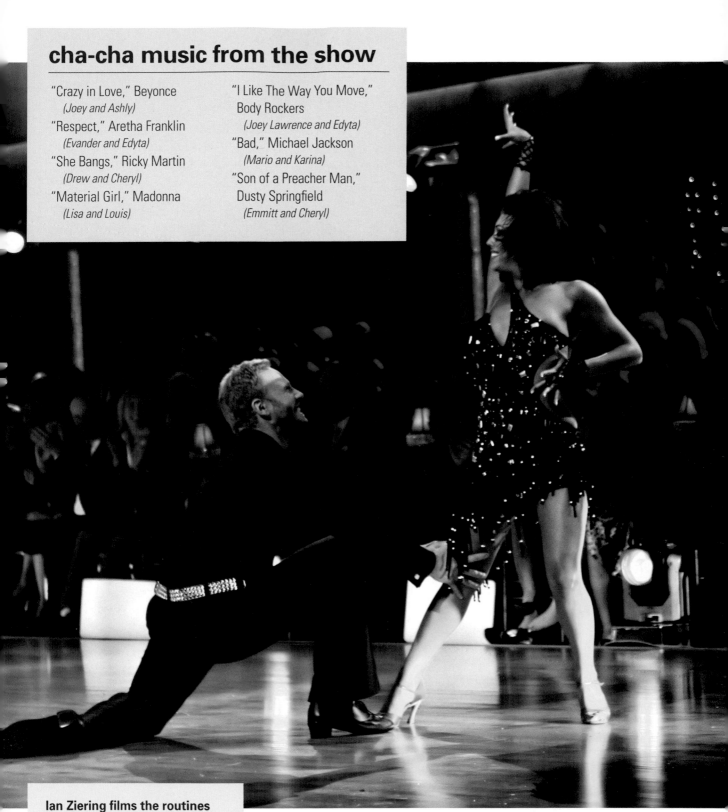

cha-cha music from the show

"Crazy in Love," Beyonce
(Joey and Ashly)

"Respect," Aretha Franklin
(Evander and Edyta)

"She Bangs," Ricky Martin
(Drew and Cheryl)

"Material Girl," Madonna
(Lisa and Louis)

"I Like The Way You Move,"
Body Rockers
(Joey Lawrence and Edyta)

"Bad," Michael Jackson
(Mario and Karina)

"Son of a Preacher Man,"
Dusty Springfield
(Emmitt and Cheryl)

Ian Ziering films the routines on his video camera and studies them at home every night.

Ian Ziering and Cheryl Burke with the perfect Cha-cha look.

cha-cha

louis van amstel's how to

- The Cha-cha is the most playful and sexy of all Latin dances, like a cat and mouse game between two lovers.

- This dance is full of nice rhythms and quick foot movements, with the judges looking for strong arm actions and good finish in the fingers.

This is a great example of Drew's so-called checked forward. It's a step we use every time we change direction from forward to backward. Even though Cheryl's weight goes further than Drew's (which is necessary) he still keeps a great posture and is capable of keeping Cheryl on her balance and not pulling her off her feet. It looks easier than it is. Very impressive!

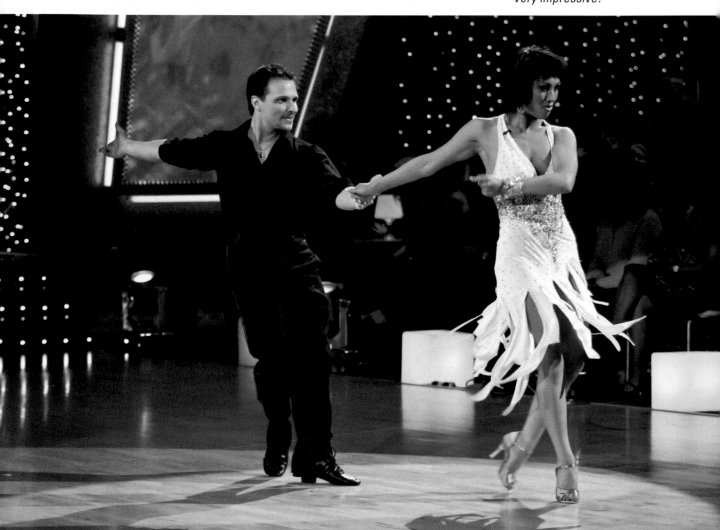

- There are lots of twists and explosive hip movements, moving the weight from one foot to the other.

- Like most other Latin dances, forward walks are taken on the balls of the feet.

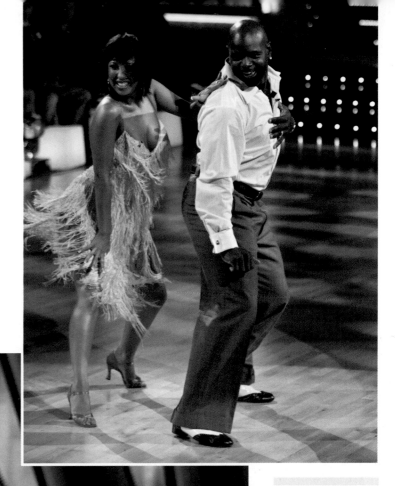

Pure joy and rhythm from Emmitt Smith and Cheryl, keeping it simple to allow Emmitt's personality and musicality to shine through.

A perfect New Yorker by Mario Lopez and Karina Smirnoff, making a complicated Cha-cha move look easy and fun.

cha-cha **45**

cha-cha
louis van amstel's how to

◆ The Cha-cha is a mostly stationary dance, with the feet turned out, rooting the couple to the floor.

◆ Basic Latin figures like the New Yorker, Hip Twist, Alamana, and Swiffles are often used by the professionals as part of their choreography.

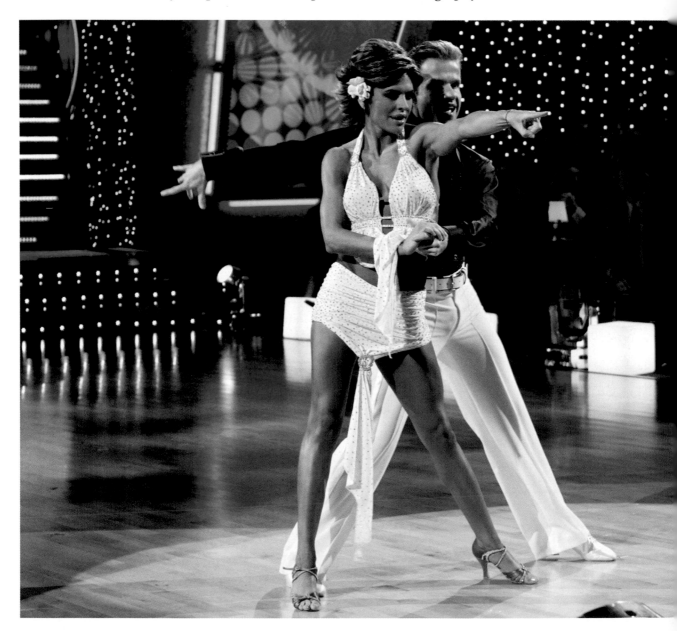

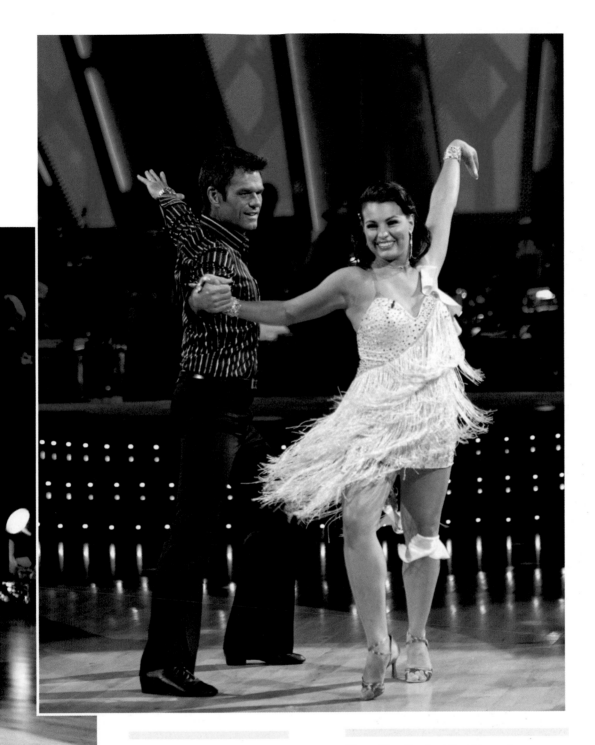

Lisa Rinna and Louis van Amstel in a playful Cha-cha mood, showing the great control she grew to master during the series.

Harry Hamlin shedding his serious reputation to have fun with his Cha-cha, showing a great arm line and twisting Ashly Costa around in lots of Swiffles.

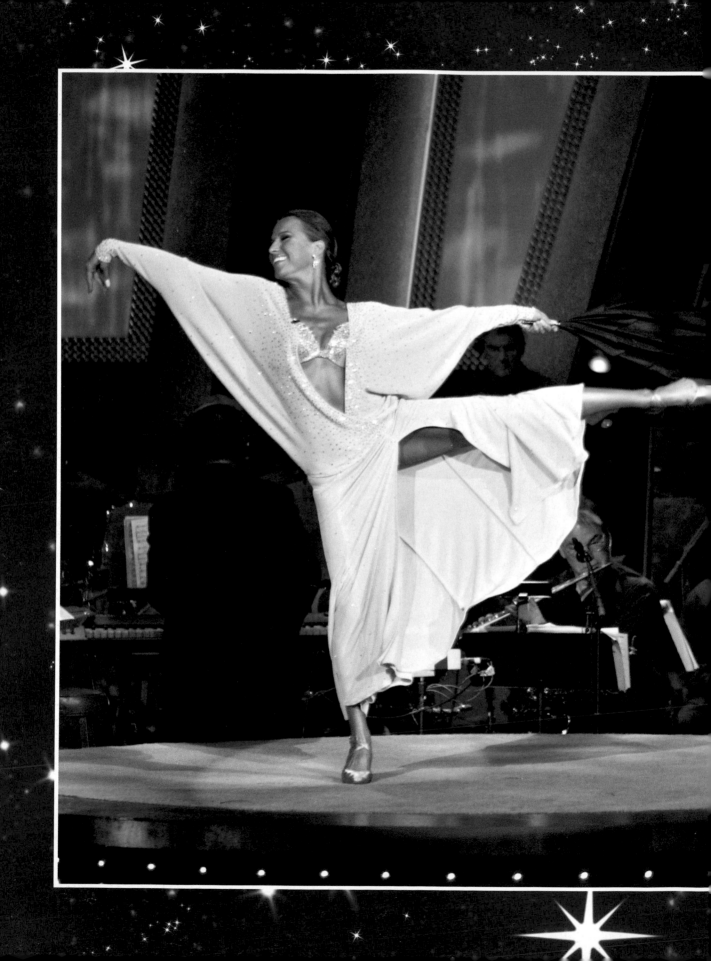

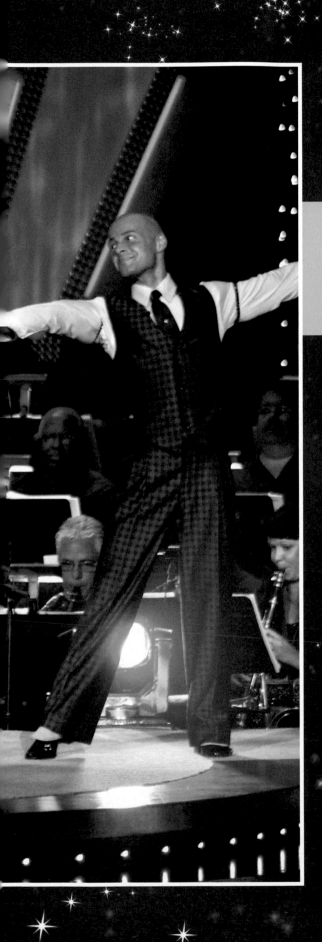

foxtrot

The epitome of sophistication and elegance, the Foxtrot evokes images of Fred Astaire and Ginger Rogers.

In 1914, when Ragtime was the dance of choice, a vaudeville actor named Harry Fox was having trouble finding women partners who could mimic the dance's tricky moves. So, he added slower steps. Soon, clientele at the Club Jardin de Danse, above the theater where Fox performed, adopted their own version of "Fox's Trot." This eventually caught the eye of Vernon and Irene Castle (a husband-and-wife dancing team), who put their own stamp on the dance, making it the graceful Foxtrot featured in the Fred Astaire movies and that we still see today.

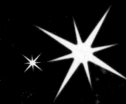

a fabulous foxtrot

Joey Lawrence and Edyta Sliwinska (Season 3, show 7)
Also seen in the *Dancing with the Stars* tour, 2006.

Having been plunged into the mortifying glare of the red light in the previous week's show, Joey and Edyta pulled out all the stops with their refined Foxtrot.

To avoid any repeat comments that their performance lacked charisma and personality, they drew inspiration from one of the most charming dancers of all, Gene Kelly.

Rehearsing on the old MGM lot, where "Singin' in the Rain" was shot, the couple was able to truly grasp the enchantment and sophistication of the dance.

The epitome of Hollywood glamour. Joey Lawrence and Edyta Sliwinska 'Singing in the Rain.'

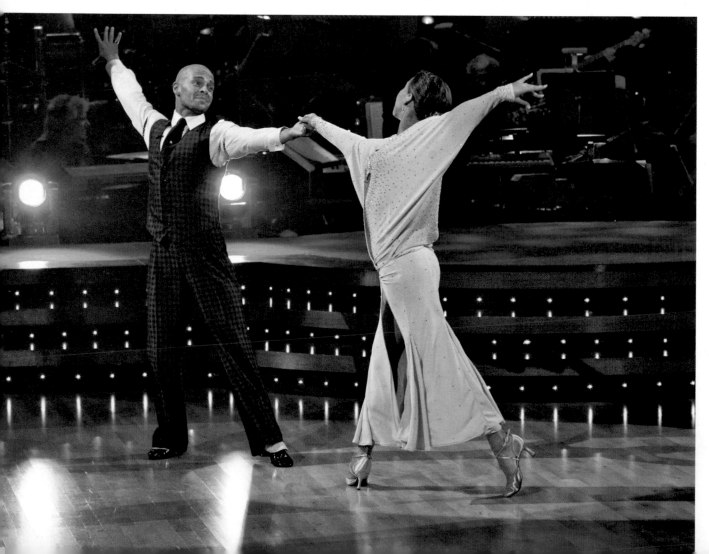

Come show night, as if possessed by Gene himself, Joey delighted the judges and scored an impressive 29 out of 30. The couple took their Foxtrot out on the road for the *Dancing* tour and received standing ovations for the performance every night. "Singin' in the Rain" is such a part of dance history that the audience recognizes the song from the first bar of music, and it was a great choice for them on the show.

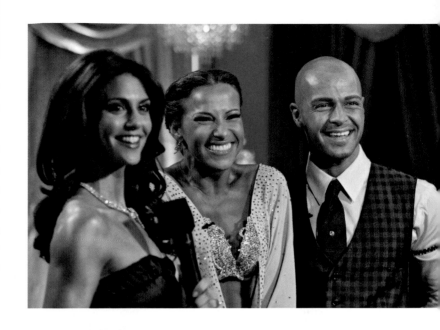

Looking pleased with a fantastic score of 29 out of 30.

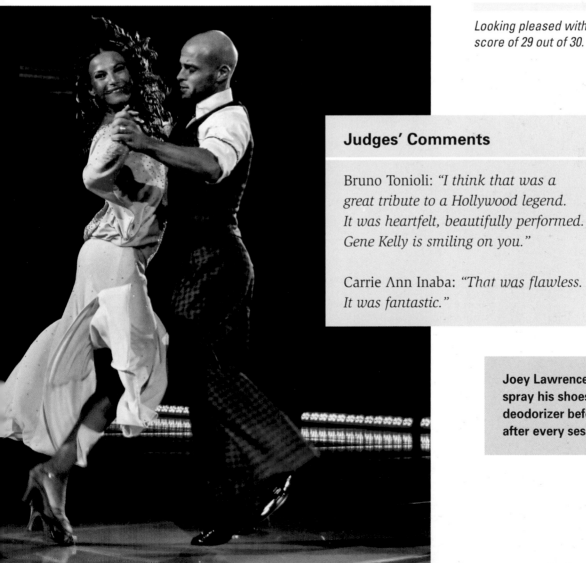

Judges' Comments

Bruno Tonioli: *"I think that was a great tribute to a Hollywood legend. It was heartfelt, beautifully performed. Gene Kelly is smiling on you."*

Carrie Ann Inaba: *"That was flawless. It was fantastic."*

the look

The Foxtrot is such an American romantic favorite. Those 1930s and 1940s design influences are perfect.

In Season four, Laila Ali's costume epitomized the Foxtrot. The rust-color silk satin charmeuse was perfect for her. The inspiration for the dress came from a red-carpet gown, which was modified to make it more practical for dancing. The ruched satin on the bustline and waist area accentuated Laila's curves. The slit in the skirt added a sexy punch to the otherwise elegant line of the gown. Lace cutwork was added and encrusted with crystals to add another dimension. Nothing moves like silk, and from the very first week Laila knew how to work that skirt!

Also in Season four Paulina Porizkova was the classic Ginger Rogers with a gorgeous updo and short waves. Her makeup was a classic matte red lip, a dramatic brow, and a clean yet dramatic eye. Paulina was the epitome of elegant Hollywood glamour.

For Shandi, it was a retro, Jessica Rabbit look. Her hair was pulled up on one side with a high, deep, sculptured wave. Makeup again was a classic red lip with a dramatic, sexy brown smoky eye perfect for the Foxtrot.

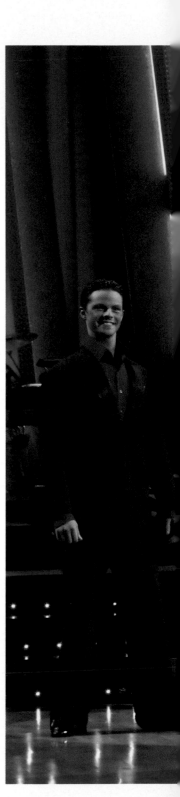

Shandi Finnessey as the embodiment of Jessica Rabbit, with partner Brian Fortuna.

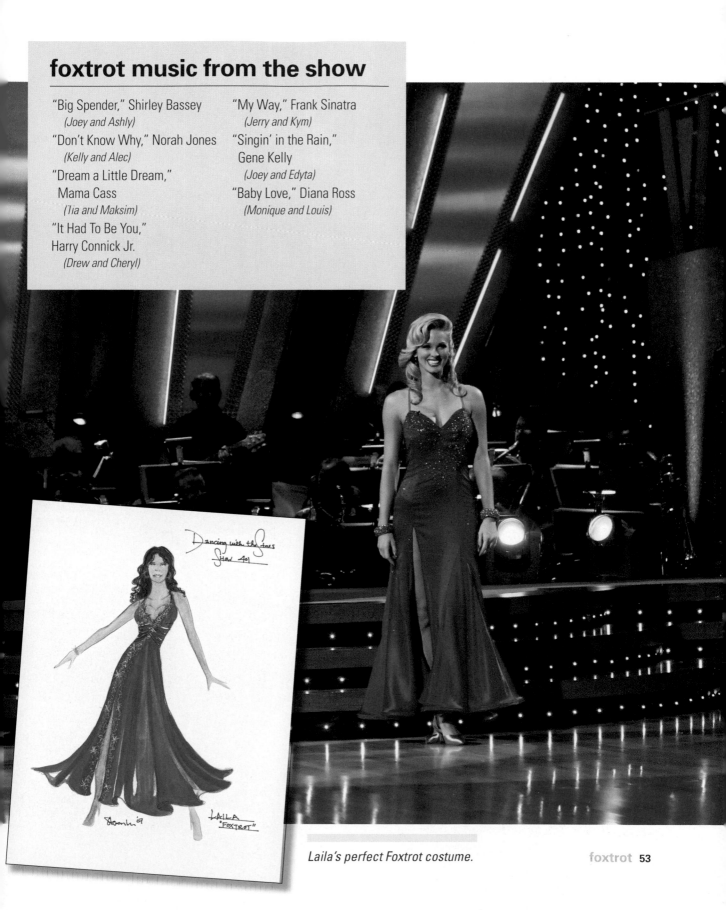

foxtrot music from the show

"Big Spender," Shirley Bassey
   (Joey and Ashly)

"Don't Know Why," Norah Jones
   (Kelly and Alec)

"Dream a Little Dream,"
   Mama Cass
   (Tia and Maksim)

"It Had To Be You,"
Harry Connick Jr.
   (Drew and Cheryl)

"My Way," Frank Sinatra
   (Jerry and Kym)

"Singin' in the Rain,"
   Gene Kelly
   (Joey and Edyta)

"Baby Love," Diana Ross
   (Monique and Louis)

Laila's perfect Foxtrot costume.

louis van amstel's how to

◆ The Foxtrot on *Dancing with the Stars* is performed in the American style, meaning the couple can be in open hold or completely unattached. The rule is that the couple must be in close hold for at least a third of the dance.

◆ The Foxtrot should be the smoothest of all ballroom dances. It should look and feel like the couple is gliding across the floor, with carefree feet mirroring each other's movements.

Just the sort of beautiful leg extension and fabulous line we came to expect from Rachel Hunter. Her professional partner Jonathan Roberts is always very clever in his ability to showcase his partner.

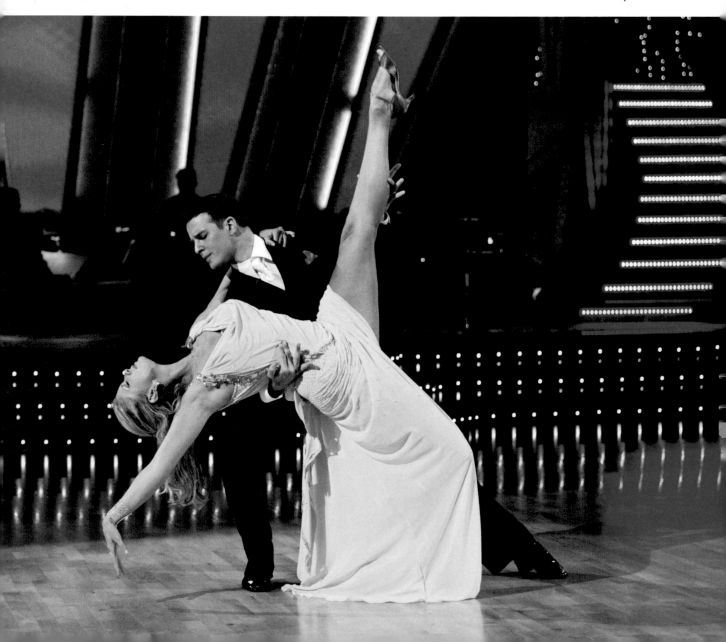

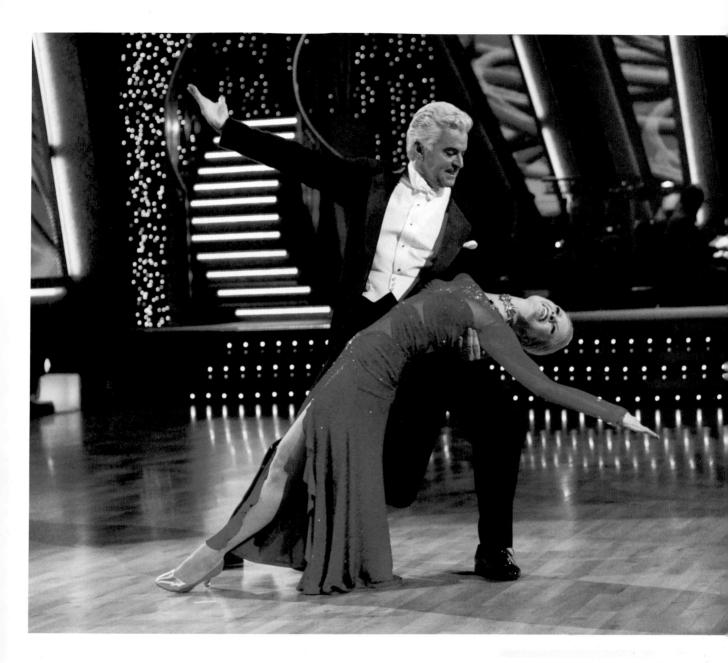

◆ Forward steps are taken over the heel for the first, then on the ball while rising up. Turning on the balls and pivoting on the heels is one of the hardest Ballroom techniques.

◆ Because there is the possibility of letting go of the hold, there is a lot more creative freedom for the dancers. However, the freedom of the Foxtrot can tempt the couple to go overboard, and so lose the character of the dance.

John O'Hurley and Charlotte always looked polished. Perfectly in character for the Foxtrot, they evoke a Fred Astaire and Ginger Rogers movie, with fantastic extension and posture.

louis van amstel's how to

◆ The ankles are working overtime to create a graceful rise and fall throughout the routine.

◆ The professionals try to use lots of graceful lines as part of their Foxtrot choreography. This tactic takes up quite some time during the performance and is mostly slow, giving the couple an opportunity to look their best and show their personality. The classic ballroom hold allows the man to perfectly communicate movements.

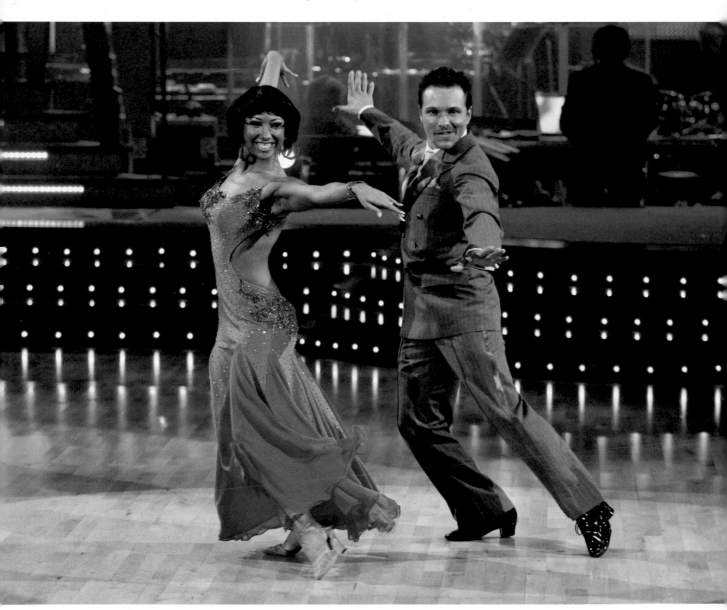

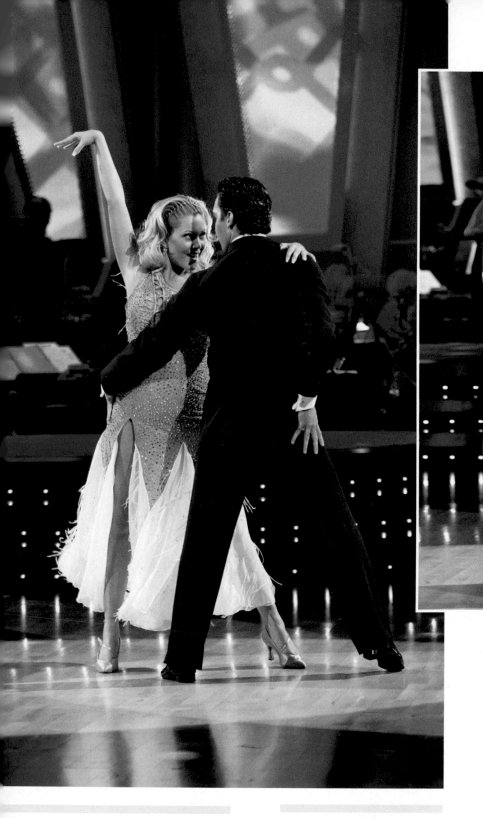

Vivica Fox and Nick Kosovich showing how romantic the Foxtrot can be and perfectly acting out their love story.

Drew and Cheryl, using all of the freedom allowed by the American-style Foxtrot, put on a highly entertaining performance.

The playful side to Foxtrot with Shanna Moakler showing great posture and extension.

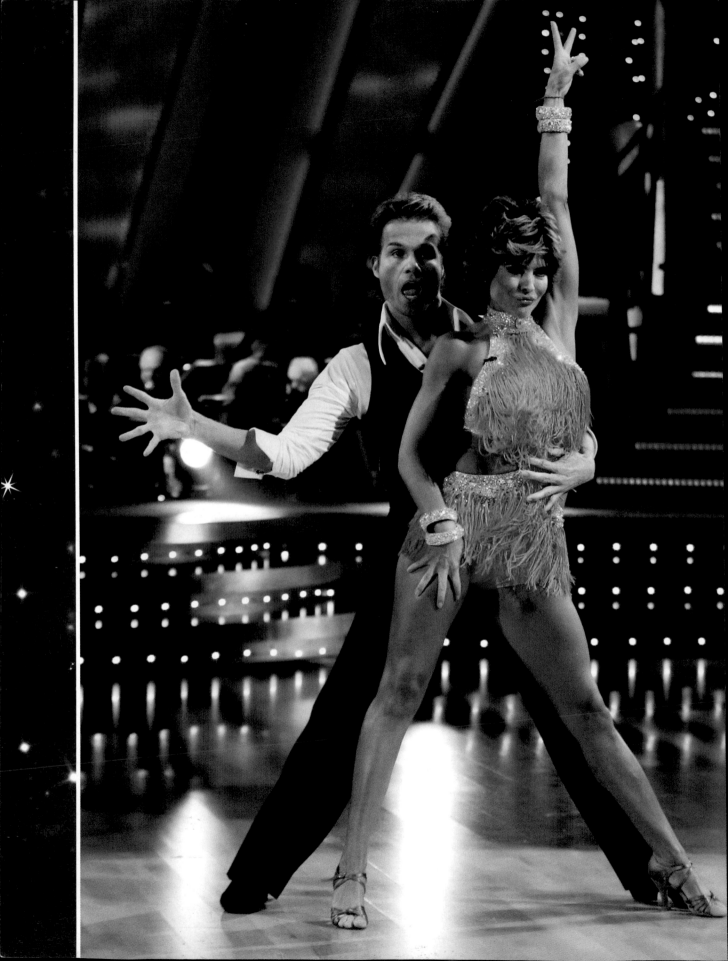

jive

A dance drawn from various origins and traditions, the Jive is fun, fast, and lively.

The most contemporary of ballroom dances, the Jive was originally an African-American dance that became the official youth dance in the jazz-crazed twenties and thirties.

GIs brought the dance over to Europe in the 1940s, where it was frowned upon because of its lively movements and spins. Nevertheless, it remained a fixture in the dance world and during the rock-and-roll fifties, gave rise to dances such as the Boogie-Woogie and the Jitterbug.

jive

a jazzy jive

Lisa Rinna and Louis van Amstel (Season 2, show 3)
Also seen in the *Dancing with the Stars* tour, 2006.

Lisa's Rumba in the previous week lacked the control that the judges were looking for, so the pressure was on to really master the Jive.

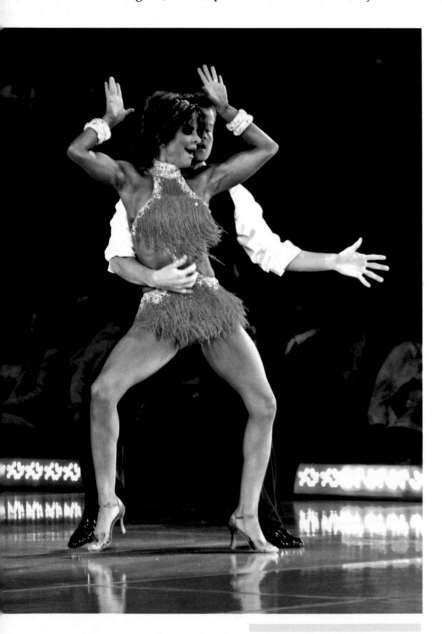

Lisa Rinna and Louis van Amstel's high energy Jive.

However, disheartened and stressed, Lisa was unable to gain the control she needed during rehearsal. The strain and frustration of training took hold. After a good cathartic cry and plenty of sound encouragement from Louis, Lisa picked herself up and dusted herself off.

"You can either lie down and roll over or you can go, 'You know what, I'm gonna meet it head-on. Bring it on!'"
—Lisa Rinna

"During the week of the Jive rehearsal I made Lisa part of the whole choreography process and she asked to make it even simpler. Lisa has so much personality that keeping the steps simple allowed her to enjoy the dance more and let her fantastic personality shine through."
—Louis van Amstel

On show night, Lisa really came out of her shell and performed the Jive as it should be performed—with energy and confidence.

Some of the studio band members used to be in Earth, Wind, and Fire.

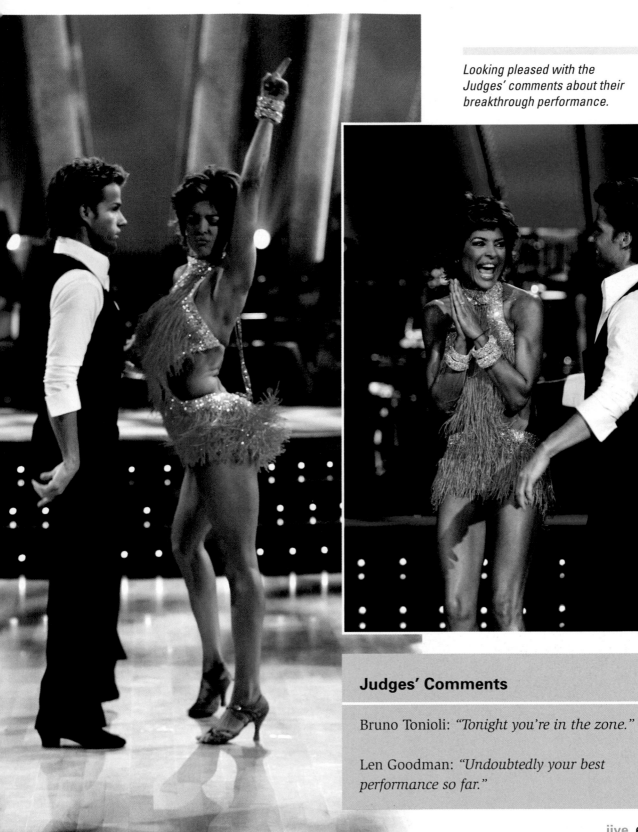

Looking pleased with the Judges' comments about their breakthrough performance.

Judges' Comments

Bruno Tonioli: *"Tonight you're in the zone."*

Len Goodman: *"Undoubtedly your best performance so far."*

jive

the look

The Jive is playful, fun, and colorful. In order to show off her new attitude, Lisa chose a fun and revealing hot pink fringe look.

Louis had a specific textured-fringe look in mind for Lisa, as texture adds much more dimension to the costume and gives so much more movement. The skirt was mounted on short shorts, which was a new concept and really allowed for Lisa to feel a lot more comfortable. After all the fringe was attached (strand by individual strand!) it was then textured up on Lisa's body. The costume designers fined-tuned the fringe the very day of the show!

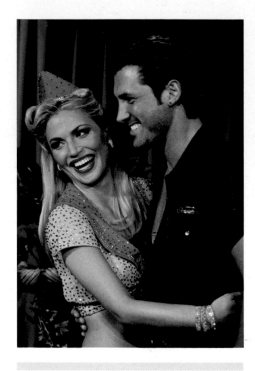

It may have come about by mistake, but Willa Ford looked stunning in her pinup girl costume, perfect for the Jive.

Willa's final costume in Season three was the result of a misunderstanding actually. Willa had given the designers an idea that she wanted to try, based on something that Christina Aguilera wore in a music video—black pants, suspenders, and a white blouse. Somehow they got got their wires crossed and instead, a classic "pin-up girl" look was designed for her, very nostalgic. It wasn't until two days later

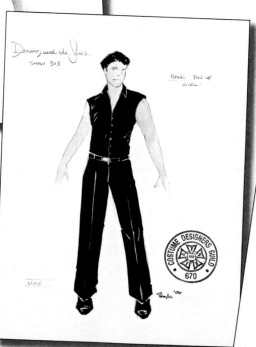

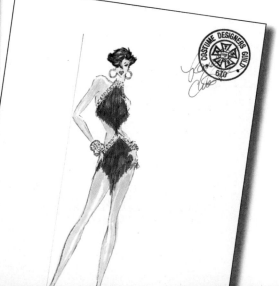

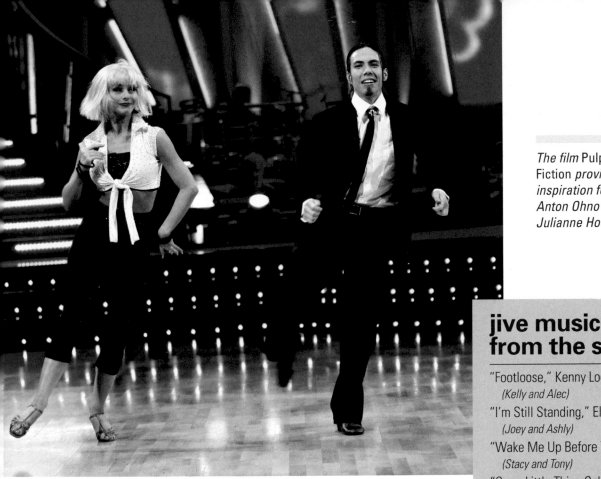

The film Pulp Fiction *provided the inspiration for Apolo Anton Ohno and Julianne Hough.*

that the mixup was discovered, and by then the costume was already in production. Nevertheless, Willa went for it.

Her hair was rolled up on the sides in a forties style to complement her sailor hat and left down in the back to soften the neckline and bounce. Makeup was classic forties mattes, with a cat's-eye liner, and a retro hot pink lip to accent the playful outfit and dance.

By the time she came onstage, she really was like a pinup girl fresh from a World War II USO club!

This look came at the perfect time for Willa, because she really felt that it was her week to be eliminated. The performance was more than enough to keep her dancing!

Julianne Hough's blonde bob in Season four was inspired by the famous dance in the movie *Pulp Fiction*. We kept it blonde to match Julianne, with a classic red lip and glowing red cheek. Apolo Anton Ohno's hair was pulled into a ponytail in homage to John Travolta.

jive
louis van amstel's how to

◆ This is the quickest of the Latin dances, with lots of kicks, flicks, and very active rebounding knees and twists, just like rock and roll. The feet flick outwards, but all movements should be precise and completed. In the same way, the arms are loose and joyous, but precise movements must extend all the way to the fingers.

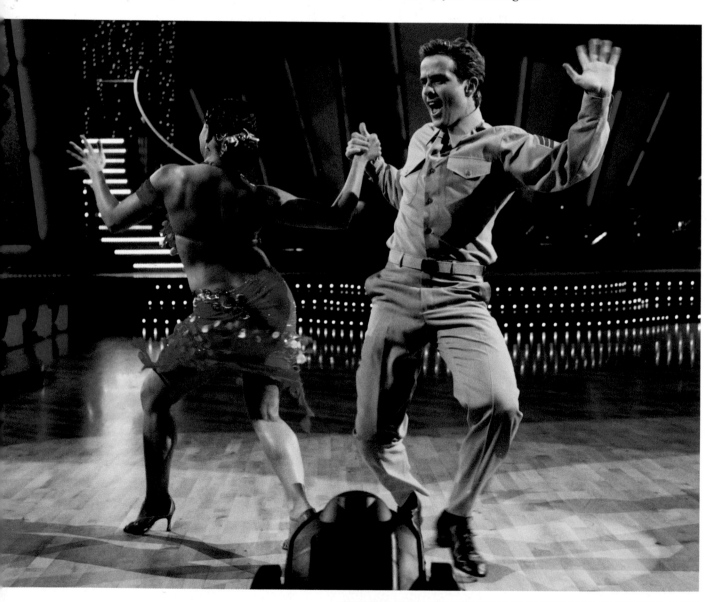

A great example of how exciting the Jive can be: Joey McIntyre shows no inhibitions with lots of crazy twists.

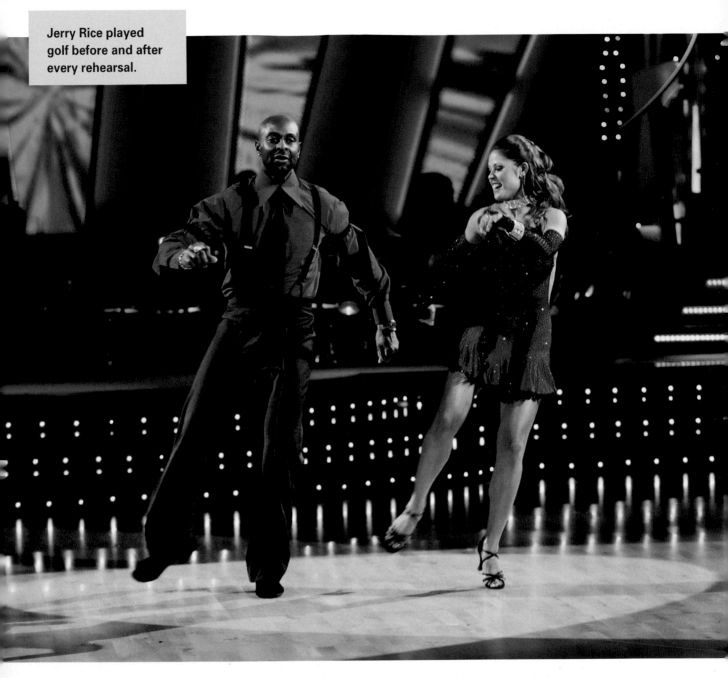

Jerry Rice played golf before and after every rehearsal.

Jerry Rice tended to look a little serious, but was able to put so much athleticism into his kicks and jumps that it was enough to create a fantastic Jive with his partner Anna Trebunskaya.

◆ Jive is also influenced by the swing dances, which have given Jive a distinct swinging action. Kicks from the hips and flicks from the knees are basic moves, and often symmetrical between the couple.

◆ Unlike the upright posture in the other Latin dances, the posture in Jive is like a weight scale or pendulum, making the swing possible. Far less rigid than in other Latin dances, the posture must adapt to the choreography.

jive

louis van amstel's how to

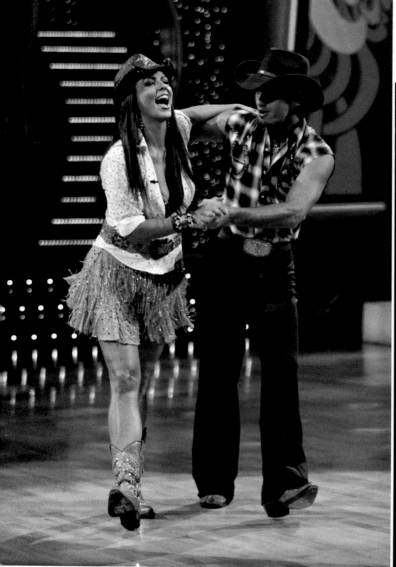

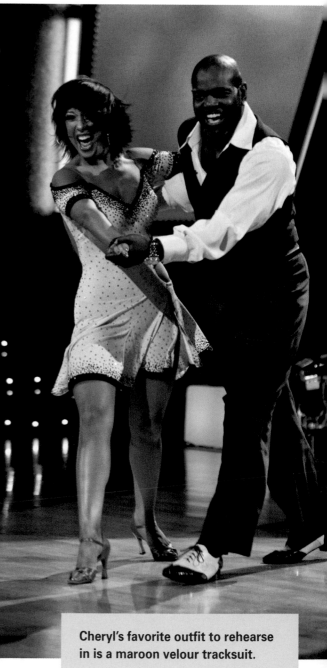

Emmitt and Cheryl having a wonderful time. These Promenade Walks are swinging like no tomorrow and are a very popular step in Jive.

Sara Evans and Tony Dovolani having a tremendous amount of fun with their Jive. Swing and country dancing are strongly related and Sara made the most of her experience. "These boots are made for Jiving!"

Cheryl's favorite outfit to rehearse in is a maroon velour tracksuit.

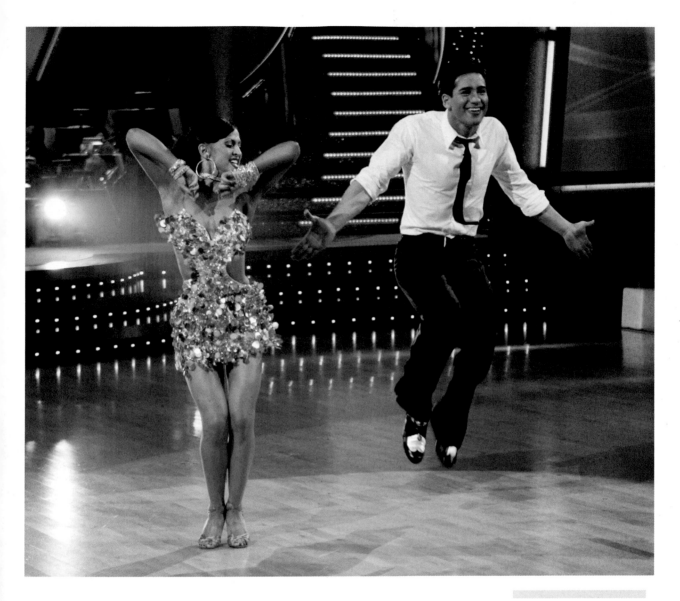

lifts

The judges criticized Joey Lawrence and Edyta during their Jive in season three for putting in lifts. So what are the rules?

Lifts are not allowed on the show until the finale, when the freestyle can include lifts. There is only one rule for the freestyle, which is that no ballroom dance is allowed, making the freestyle difficult to choreograph, and yet an interesting challenge at the same time.

Although putting lifts in a routine is more attractive and entertaining for the viewers, it can be very risky and dangerous for the celebrities who have no previous experience of lifting. Someone could get badly injured, which would just not be worth the risk. The move also gives the physically stronger competitors an unfair advantage. If the dancer does a solo cartwheel or handstand, this is not considered a lift. It is only considered a lift if one partner supports the other partner who has both feet off the ground.

High energy Jiving by Mario Lopez and Karina Smirnoff. See how high Mario has jumped, displaying a key characteristic of Jive.

jive **67**

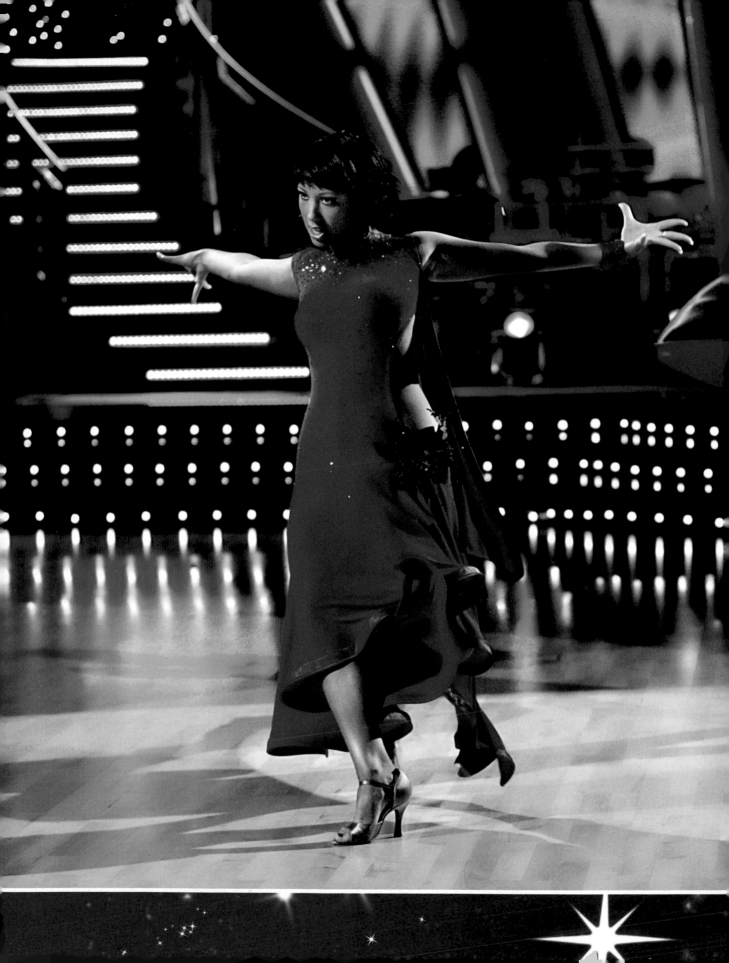

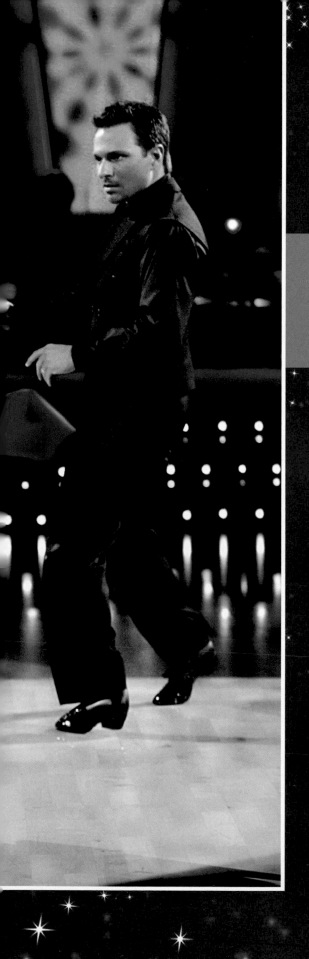

paso doble

In this ultimate expression of machismo, the man plays the brave matador and the woman plays the cape and any other roles.

A male-dominated dance that originated in Spain, the Paso Doble represents the traditional bullfight. The man plays the part of the matador, while the woman dons various hats as either the bull, the cape, or another matador or dancer.

The dance became popular in France in the 1930s and very soon the rest of the ballroom-dancing world.

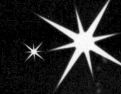

paso doble

a phenomenal paso doble

Drew Lachey and Cheryl Burke (Season 2, show 4)
Also seen on the *Dancing with the Stars* tour, 2006.

As winner of Season two, Drew was steadily impressive throughout the competition. So the real work lay in having to live up to the standards that he and his partner, Cheryl, set each week.

By week four it was time for the ultimate challenge, and what better way to conquer this challenge than to dance the intense Paso Doble.

Drew Lachey and Cheryl Burke in the heat of their passionate Paso Doble.

The iconic "Thriller" choreography. "Thriller" became one of the most popular performances on the first Dancing with the Stars *tour.*

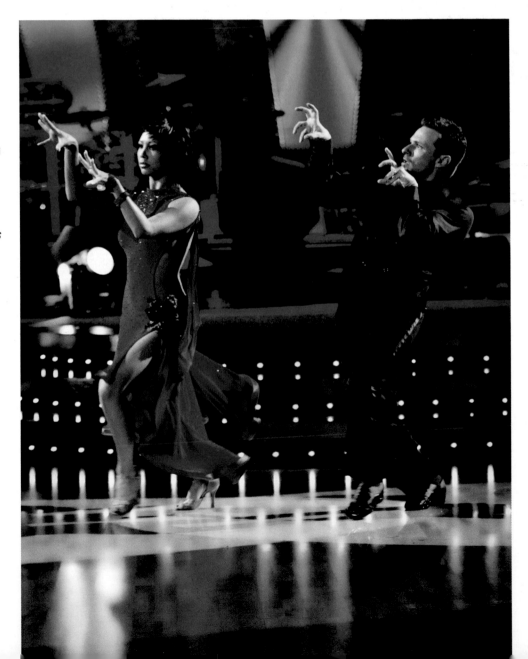

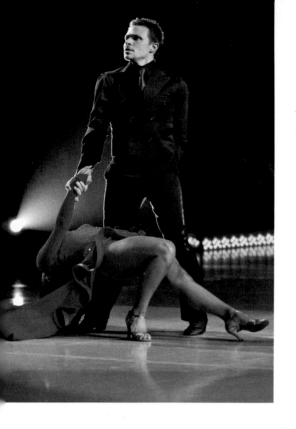

"The Paso was a bittersweet dance for me. It was a lot of work. I really had to transform myself. Physically. Personality-wise. . . . Everything we had done up to that point was a little more fun and light. But the first time I did it, I didn't quite get the scores I was hoping for. They said my shoulders were up, but when we redid it for the final, I was able to focus on my shoulders, keeping them down. Taking what the judges just said and implementing that into my performance again. You know, it was just kind of like this great feeling of satisfaction. You got the three tens pop up. That was great. That was a great moment to be able to take a dance that wasn't perfect and, at least in the judges' eyes, make it perfect. That was a sense of accomplishment."

—Drew Lachey, talking about his Paso Doble "Thriller"

Not an intimidating person by nature, Drew had trouble adopting the posture and the arrogant attitude of the matador. So they brought a real matador into the dance studio, to instruct and advise on key moves and temperaments.

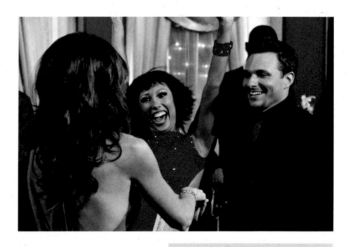

By the night of the show, Drew's matador pride took hold, and to an electrifying rendition of Michael Jackson's "Thriller," he and Cheryl undoubtedly "thrilled" the judges.

Judges' Comments

Carrie Ann Inaba: *"The Paso Doble is all about passion, power, being in control on the dance floor. You dominated the dance floor."*

Bruno Tonioli: *"You have become a truly believable leading man. Strong, powerful, commanding, in control. You have achieved greatness."*

Cheryl celebrating the Judges' triple ten score in the finale.

The couple scored 28 out of 30, and then refined and perfected the dance for the finale, where they scored a triple 10.

paso doble

the look

As the dance was so close to Mario's heritage, he was very specific about how he wanted to look for the Paso Doble. He asked to emulate the style of Antonio Banderas in *El Mariachi* because he was dancing to a song from the movie. A glistening scorpion embroidered on the back of his bolero jacket was a perfect addition to the ensemble. Karina Smirnoff's golden yellow dress complemented the embellishment and was a real hit, despite causing a few problems during rehearsals (trips and rips!) Nevertheless, with hurried adjustments, what the viewers saw on show night truly enhanced their excellent performance.

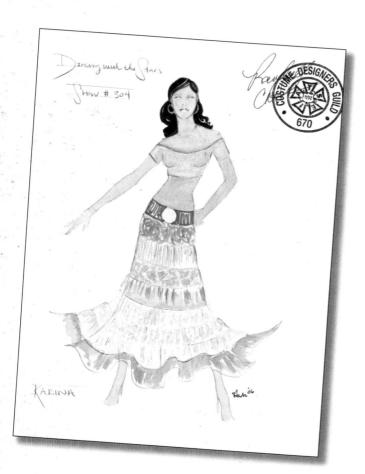

It was the traditional look for Lisa; her hair was darkened with temporary bleach mousses with added hairpieces to give her length to be pulled back in a low bun. Finishing touches were a traditional flower and extremely tanned skin with dramatic eyes and strong eyebrows and nude lip.

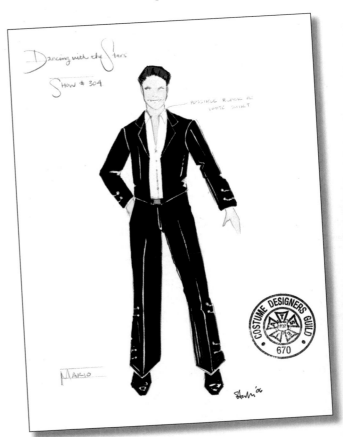

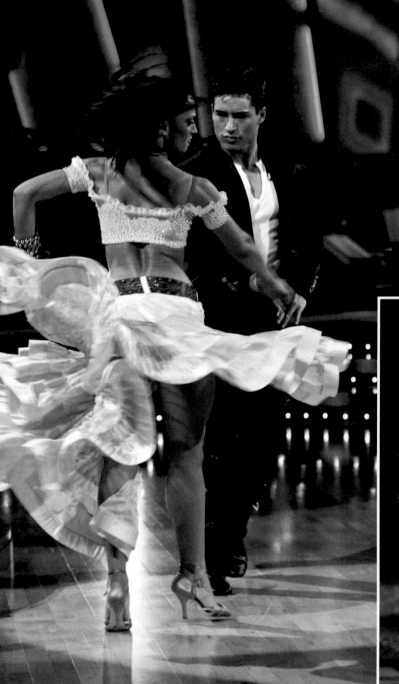

Mario Lopez and Karina Smirnoff,
a classic Paso look.

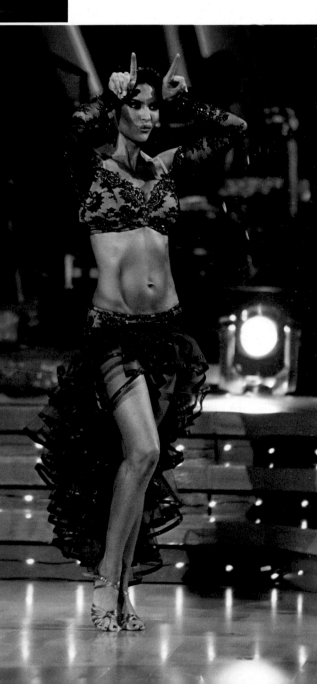

Lisa Rinna ready to charge!

paso doble
louis van amstel's how to

◆ The most aggressive and powerful dance should not lose its passionate energy. Many times this dance is misunderstood and made to look too angry.

◆ There should be strong eye contact and tension, evoking either the bullfight or Flamenco character.

Dancing with the Stars is responsible for a wedding. Professional dancer Ashly DelGrosso met her future husband Mike Costa on Season one when he was the producer assigned to film her and Joey McIntyre! They married in 2006.

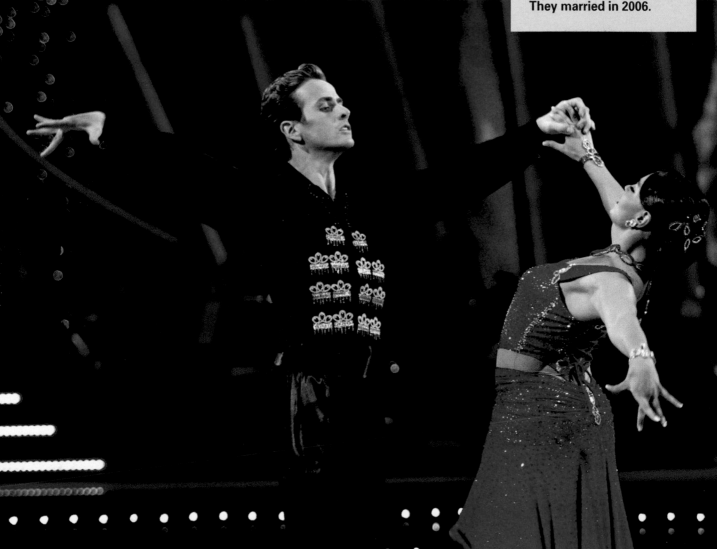

Joey McIntyre as the matador and Ashly Costa as his cape.

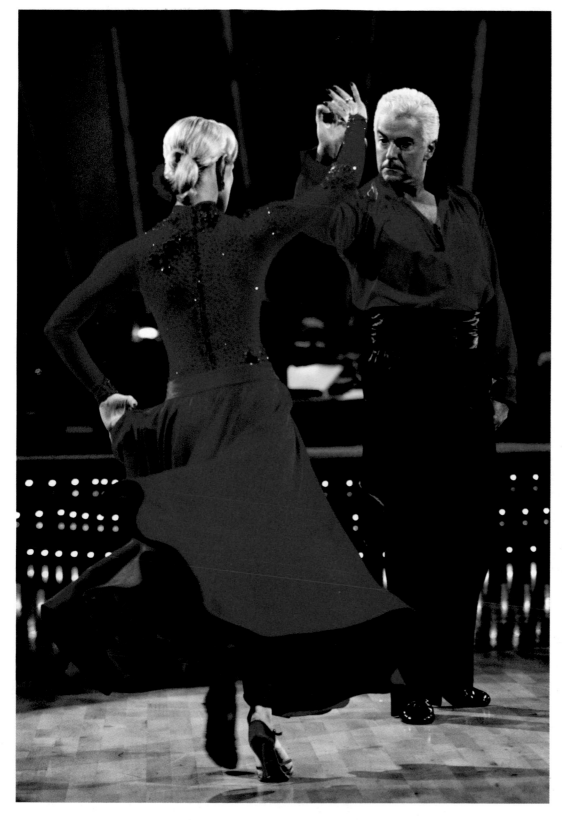

Great posture and intensity from John and Charlotte, who despite being stronger at the ballroom dances, excelled with this performance.

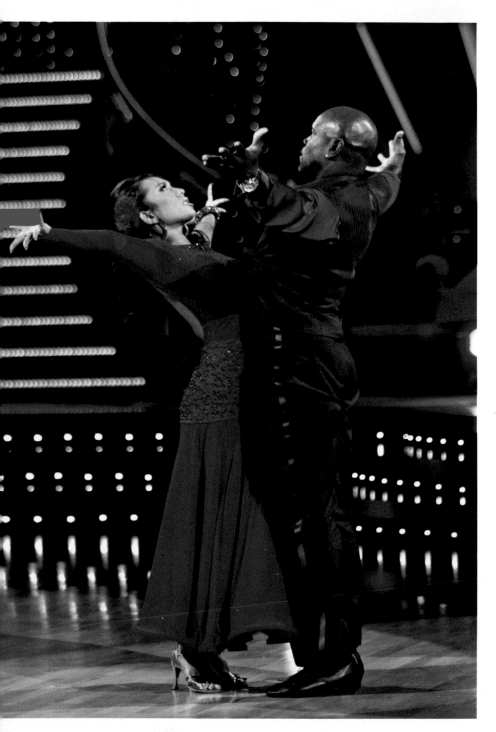

- Unlike the other Latin dances, the walks in Paso Doble are marching steps and taken over the heel. Flamenco walks in Paso are lunges taken over the balls of the feet.

- A high degree of flexibility is required, with both partners bending into extreme lines, flexing through the spine.

- The arms emphasize the strength of the matador and the flexibility of the woman, with the feet often telling a story by attracting the attention of the bull.

Another fantastic posture and arm movement from Emmitt and Cheryl. In full contact here, they are preparing for a basic movement, with Emmitt displaying all of his strength as matador.

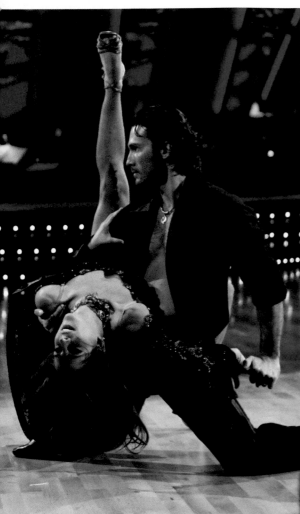

A perfect example of the bullfight influence in the Paso Doble. Kelly Monaco is the cape, draped over the knees of matador Alec Mazo at the end of the fight. Kelly is showing incredible leg extension here.

Passion, tension, and focus between Emmitt and Cheryl. A perfect posture, so simple and yet so expressive.

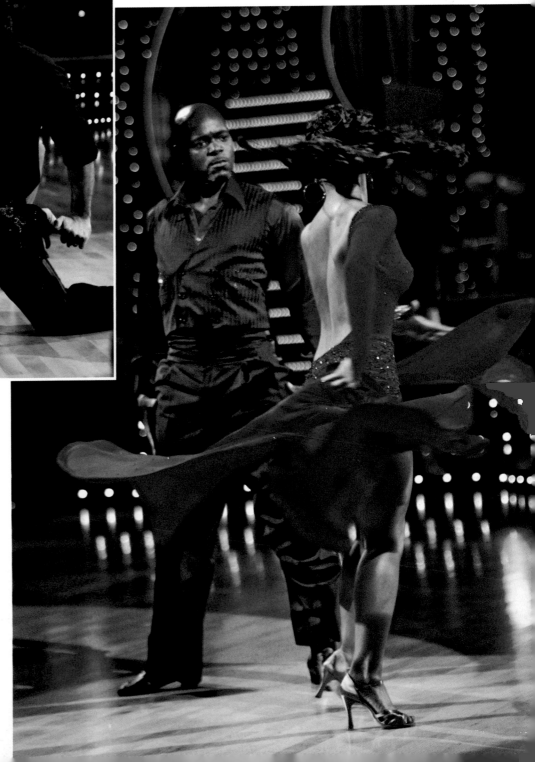

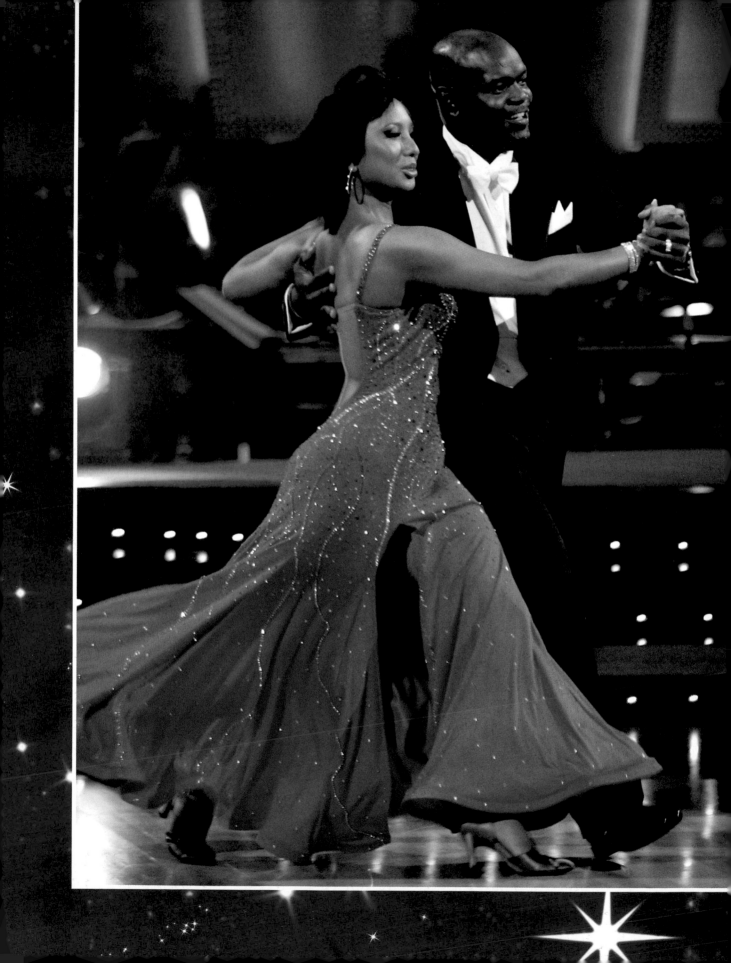

quickstep

This fast and vibrant dance is a favorite of ballroom dancers worldwide.

In the 1920s, when the Foxtrot was the most popular dance, bands started to play the music faster, so that it was hard for all but the most experienced dancers to keep up. Thus, the Quickstep was conceived, incorporating elements of the Charleston (another dance craze).

In 1927, it was introduced into competitions by English dancers Frank Ford and Molly Spain. It became incredibly popular and evolved into a zestful dance of seemingly endless possibilities.

quickstep

a quality quickstep
Emmitt Smith and Cheryl Burke (Season 3, show 2)

Having started the competition with a fantastic Cha-cha, Emmitt was looking like he might be the surprise of the competition, and the Quickstep put this beyond doubt. As he and Cheryl had struggled in training and tired from the commute to Emmitt's home in Dallas, the odds were stacked against them, but like the true champions they went on to become, they were able to put in a great performance, scoring 8, 8, 8.

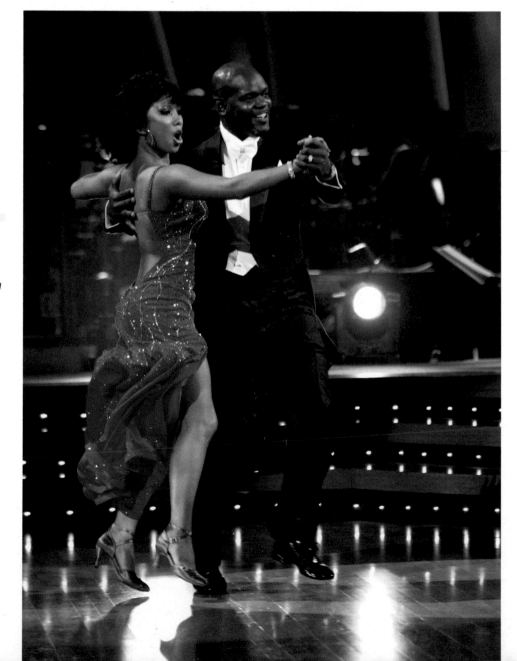

"I designed this dance to let Emmitt have fun, to modernize the dance and to prove to America that Emmitt Smith is indeed the epitome of everything Quickstep."
—Cheryl Burke

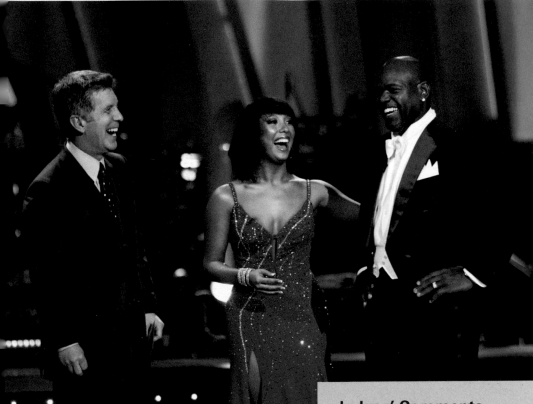

Emmitt looking surprised but pleased with his new nickname "Twinkle Toes."

Physically Emmitt is built for rushing yards and winning Superbowls, which makes his mastery of the Quickstep all the more impressive. The fact that Carrie Ann named him "Twinkle Toes" was quite extraordinary.

Judges' Comments

Carrie Ann Inaba: *"I hope you don't take this the wrong way: Would, do you mind if I call you Twinkle Toes?"*

Bruno Tonioli: *"You really come equipped with a natural license to thrill . . . it was absolutely delightful."*

Len Goodman: *"A great performance, well done."*

"The pressure to win was great—I had to beat Jerry Rice. I mean, from a fan perspective, Jerry had set the mark high, so the question was, Can I beat Jerry? Winning was my number one motivation. My number one motivation was to win."

—Emmitt Smith, talking about his motivation to perform

Emmitt Smith used to eat at Mastro's Steakhouse after every show. His favorite dish is buttermilk cake.

quickstep

the look

The fantastic costumes and hair and makeup designs made the Quickstep truly shine. Edyta was in her lovely nothingness, in a dress that was barely there. The costume designers have challenges weekly, trying to find ways to conceal the dancers' microphone packs, as they all wear them during their performances. Edyta's mic pack was right in the center back of her skirt, right at the upper edge.

Because the Quickstep is full of hops, skips, and jumps (it's quite bouncy), her skirt kept slipping down, exposing just a bit too much of Edyta. The designers were quite busy trying to anchor not only the mic pack but also that skirt so that it didn't reveal more of Edyta than was planned.

Edyta's hair was softly pulled back from the bottom and beautifully rolled upward across the whole back of the neck to create a classic red-carpet feel. Makeup was kept simple and beautiful, to complement the rest of the ensemble.

Edyta puts the dress through its paces, showing the challenge of building beautiful costumes that can also stand up to the rigors of dancing.

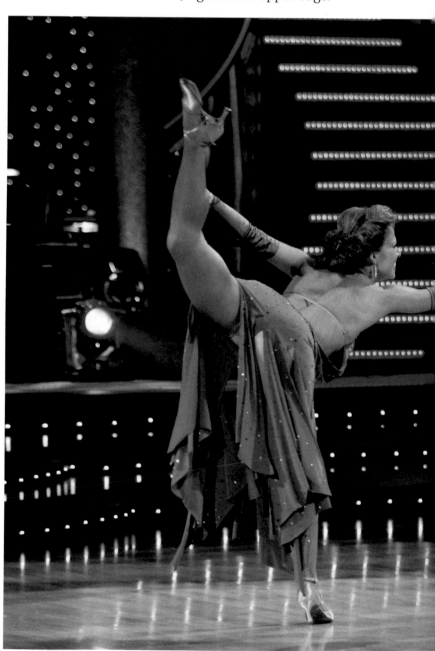

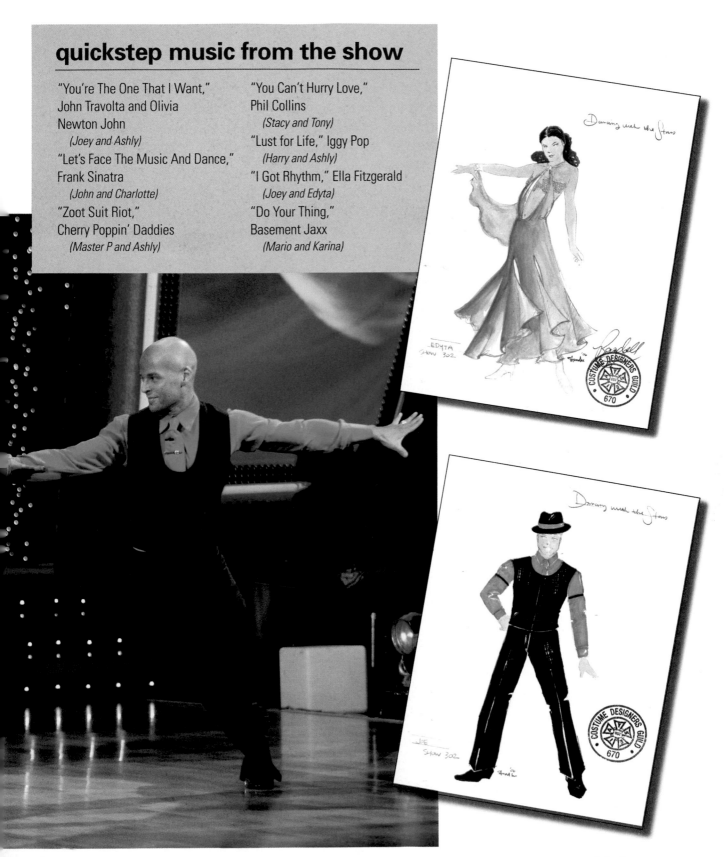

quickstep music from the show

"You're The One That I Want,"
John Travolta and Olivia
Newton John
  (Joey and Ashly)

"Let's Face The Music And Dance,"
Frank Sinatra
  (John and Charlotte)

"Zoot Suit Riot,"
Cherry Poppin' Daddies
  (Master P and Ashly)

"You Can't Hurry Love,"
Phil Collins
  (Stacy and Tony)

"Lust for Life," Iggy Pop
  (Harry and Ashly)

"I Got Rhythm," Ella Fitzgerald
  (Joey and Edyta)

"Do Your Thing,"
Basement Jaxx
  (Mario and Karina)

quickstep

louis van amstel's how to

◆ As its name suggests, the Quickstep is the quickest dance in the ballroom and should be an exciting spectacle.

◆ Fast foot patterns are used with lots of jumping, interchanged with smooth swinging figures to create a great mixture of dynamics. A skipping dance with lots of running steps.

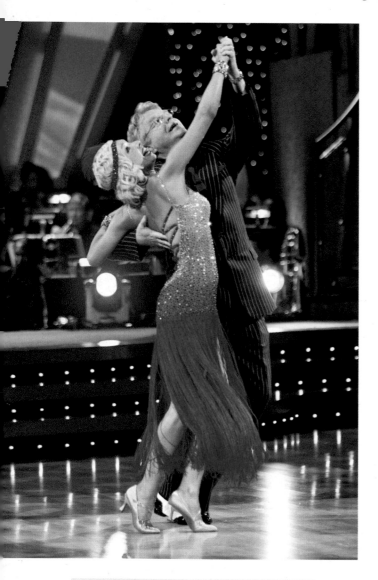

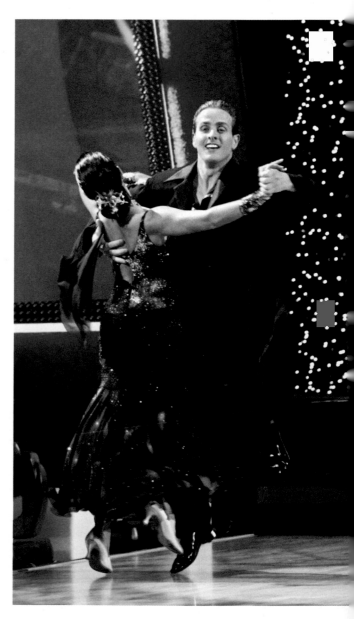

Jerry again showing his ability to entertain and delight. This shot depicts a fun and different way to perform the Charleston Quickstep while still retaining the close hold, showcasing clever choreography by Kym.

- Unlike the Waltz and the Foxtrot, the Quickstep is danced in the international style, meaning the couple has to stay in close hold and in touch with each other from the hips to the mid-torso. This is incredibly hard to learn in such a short space of time on the show, but when mastered it is beautiful to watch two people move as one.

- An open routine is only allowed in the first and last ten seconds of the performance. The remainder of the performance must be completed in the classic ballroom hold.

- The Quickstep derives from the Charleston and was always performed upright, due to the corsets and dresses worn in that era. The opposite of the lindy hop from the same period, which was anything but upright!

Joey McIntyre and Ashly Costa fizzing with energy, with the jumps and speed that characterize the Quickstep.

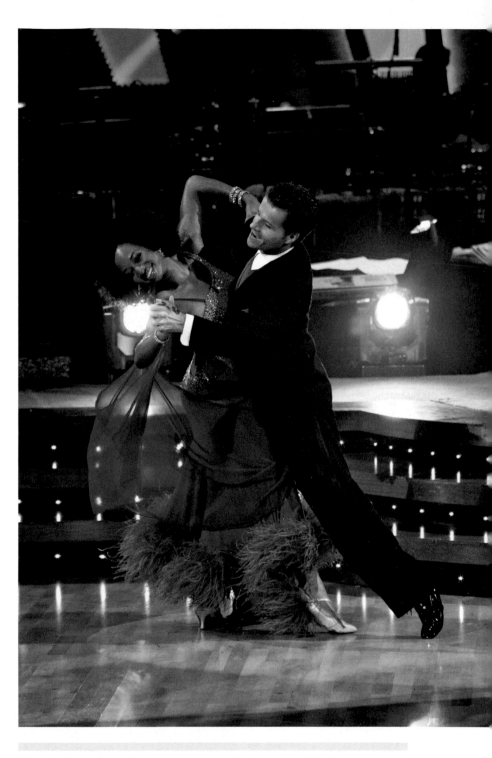

What a shame that Monique stepped on her feathers! But like a pro she managed to keep going as if nothing had happened. In this picture she shows beautiful posture, while keeping the bodies in contact.

louis van amstel's how to

◆ The Quickstep is taken forward on the heel on the first step, and on the ball on the second and third, with a slow, quick, quick timing. The feet should be light on the floor, with weightless pivot turns.

◆ The Quickstep has lots of rise and fall, but it is important not to rise too soon and too long, otherwise you can't keep up with the speed and will fly off the dance floor.

Again, the high energy of Mario and Karina is obvious, although they were heavily criticized by the judges for too much open work. Here, they show the influence of the Charleston in their Quickstep.

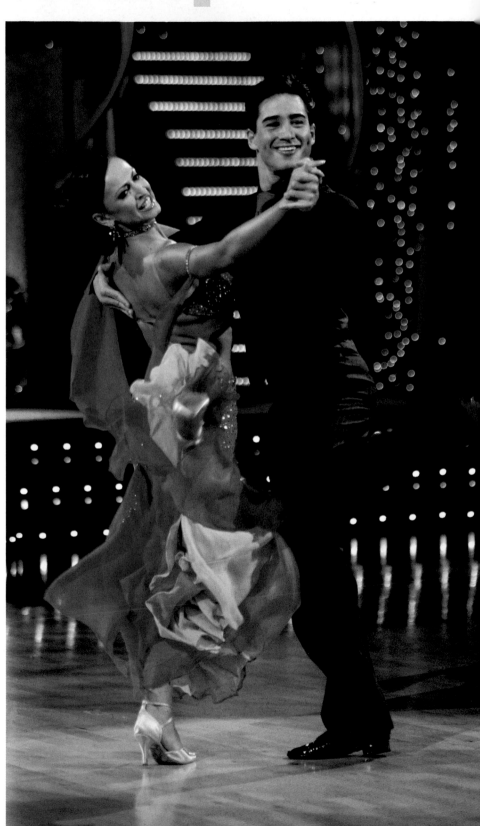

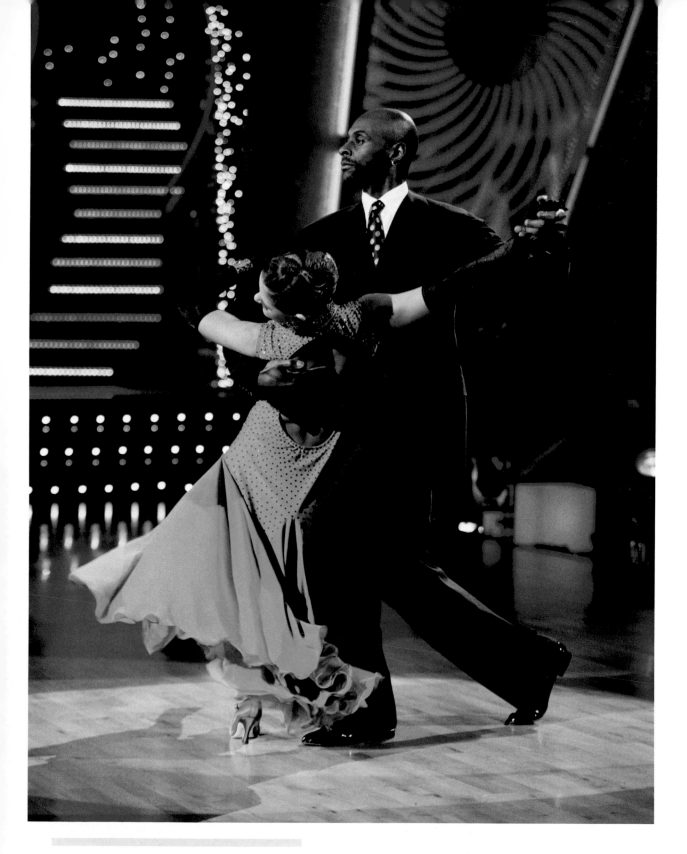

Despite being twisted in a left whisk, Jerry manages to maintain great posture, a difficult line to create with all that speed.

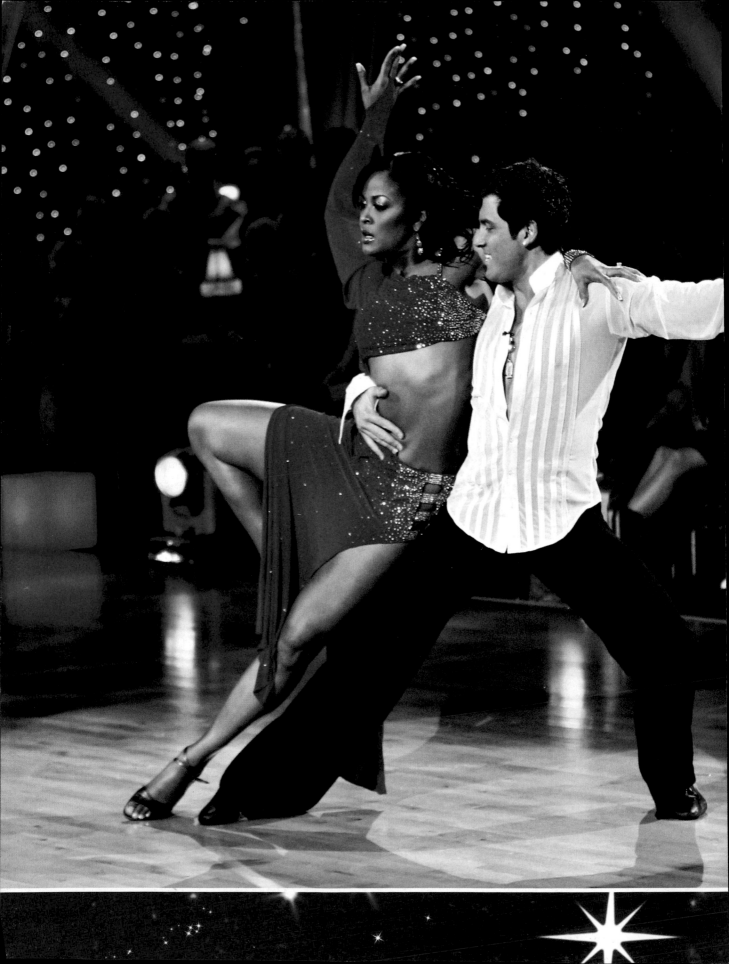

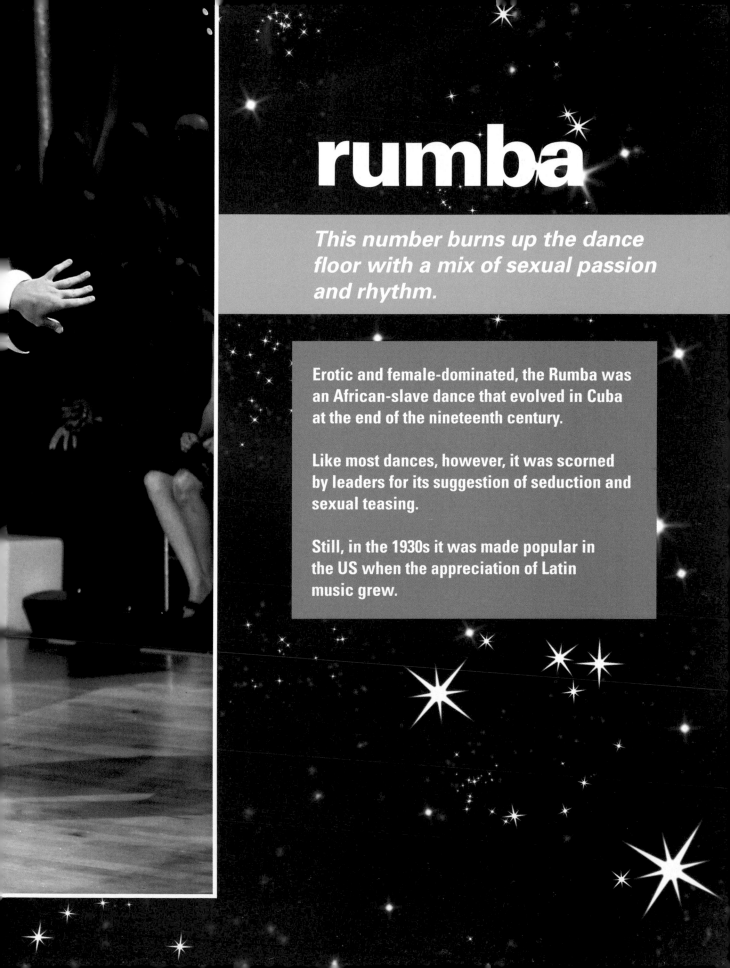

rumba

This number burns up the dance floor with a mix of sexual passion and rhythm.

Erotic and female-dominated, the Rumba was an African-slave dance that evolved in Cuba at the end of the nineteenth century.

Like most dances, however, it was scorned by leaders for its suggestion of seduction and sexual teasing.

Still, in the 1930s it was made popular in the US when the appreciation of Latin music grew.

rumba

a romantic rumba
Laila Ali and Maksim Chmerkovskiy (Season 4, show 5)

In the previous week, boxer Laila left the judges cold with her performance in the Paso Doble, scoring 7, 7, 7.

"I'm used to being on top. I'm used to being number one."—Laila Ali

Nevertheless, the disenchantment didn't stop her. It only fueled the fire and she was ready to take it to the next level.

Laila Ali making quite an entrance for her Rumba.

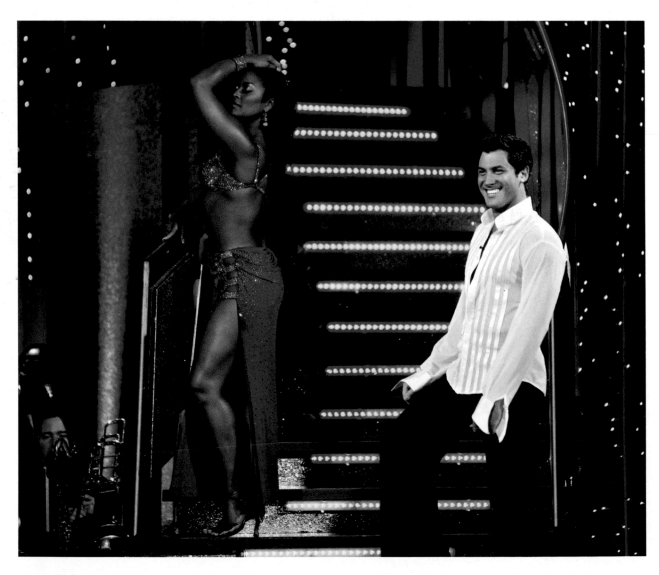

The judges wanted Laila to add passion and energy to her dancing, and the Rumba was the perfect choice to do just that.

Because the Rumba is an incredibly sensual and erotic dance, Laila's intention was to let her hair down (literally!) and really sex it up. However, out of respect to her fiancé, she had him come to rehearsals to make sure the number wasn't too x-rated.

And it wasn't. On show night, Laila pleased both her fiancé and the judges with a gorgeous performance that brought her back to where she wanted to be—on top.

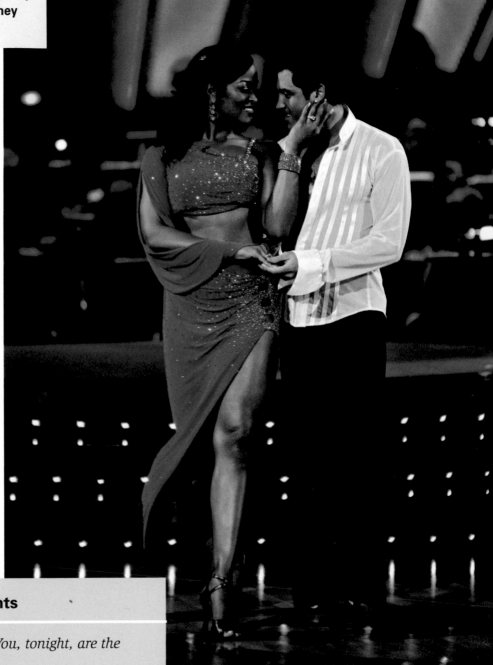

Laila and Maks treading a fine line between portraying the romance of the Rumba and upsetting Laila's fiancé!

Judges' Comments

Carrie Ann Inaba: *"You, tonight, are the comeback kid."*

Len Goodman: *"That was your best performance of the season."*

Bruno Tonioli: *"That was luscious Laila back in smoldering form. So sexy."*

rumba

the look

Edyta was inspiring and inspired with this Rumba costume. She wears so little so well! She chose to wrap herself in a ten-yard silk satin "sheet" with one leg and one bare shoulder exposed. The skirt was heavily trimmed with rhinestones, which caused some trouble in rehearsal, but by showtime only helped to intensify the provocative dance.

The look is Latin yet soft and seductive. Stacy Keibler had a half-up hairstyle with an off-center part and a long, soft, flowy fringe framing her neck and shoulders. The makeup was glowing and soft with a nude lip and smoky eye.

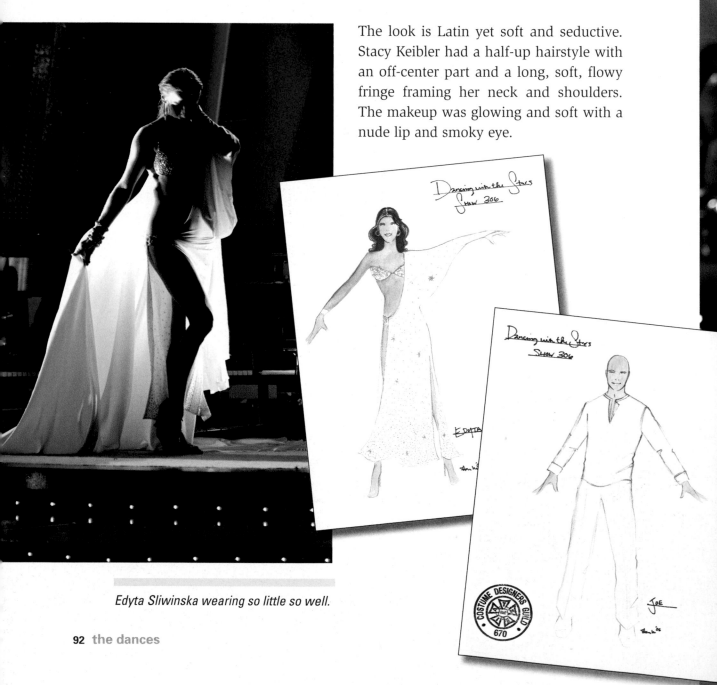

Edyta Sliwinska wearing so little so well.

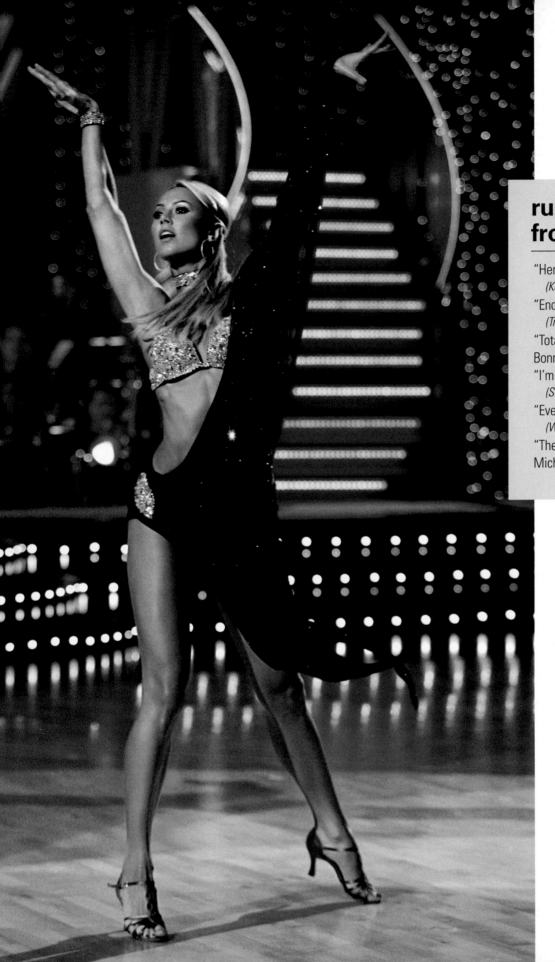

rumba music from the show

"Hero," Enrique Iglesias
 (Kelly and Alec)
"Endless Love," Lionel Richie
 (Trista and Louis)
"Total Eclipse of the Heart,"
Bonnie Tyler *(Drew and Cheryl)*
"I'm Like a Bird," Nelly Furtado
 (Stacy and Tony)
"Every Breath You Take," Police
 (Willa and Maksim)
"They Way You Look Tonight,"
Michael Bublé *(Mario and Karina)*

*Stacy Keibler
with a classic
Rumba look.*

rumba

louis van amstel's how to

- The Rumba should include lots of sensual hip action and a seductive energy between the two dancers.

- If the couple decides to interpret the Rumba in a more abstract way, the energy can become less romantic and more spiritual.

The slow pace of the Rumba allows time for the dancers to create fabulous lines, like this picture-perfect line of Drew and Cheryl.

◆ Forward walks are taken on the balls of the feet, and since the Rumba is the slowest of all Latin dances, leg action and extensions are very important in showing beautiful legs and balance. Weight shifts from leg to leg, thrusting the hips from side to side, with the unstressed leg extended fully.

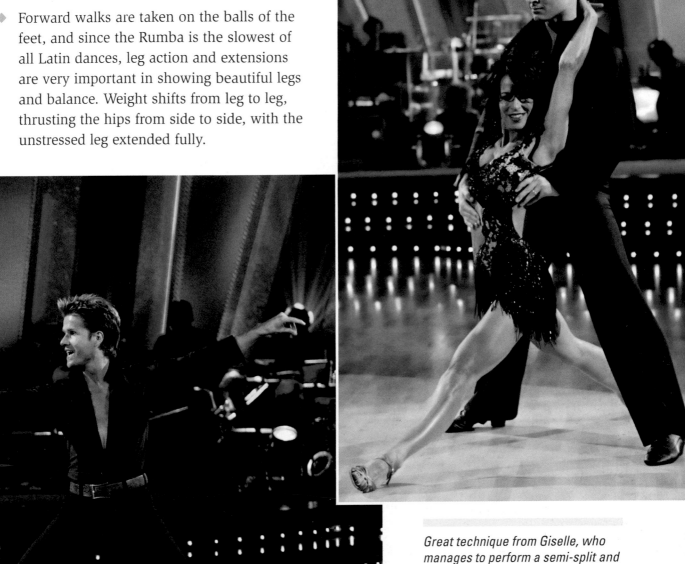

Great technique from Giselle, who manages to perform a semi-split and full arm extension while displaying such sensuality in her face.

Lisa showing fabulous leg and arm extension and a great sensual Rumba character.

rumba

louis van amstel's how to

◆ The Rumba is a great opportunity to display beautiful lines and the flexibility of your partner.

◆ The Rumba figures such as Sliding Doors, Cucaracha, and Hip Twists have been used by all of the professionals on the show.

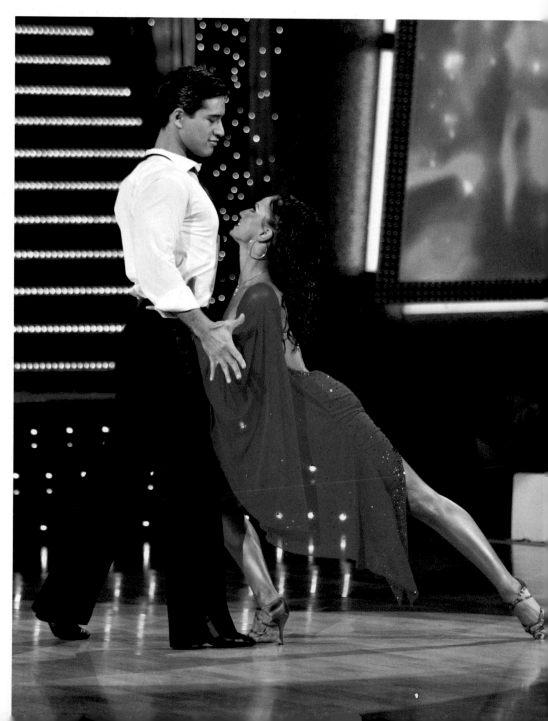

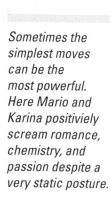

Sometimes the simplest moves can be the most powerful. Here Mario and Karina positiviely scream romance, chemistry, and passion despite a very static posture.

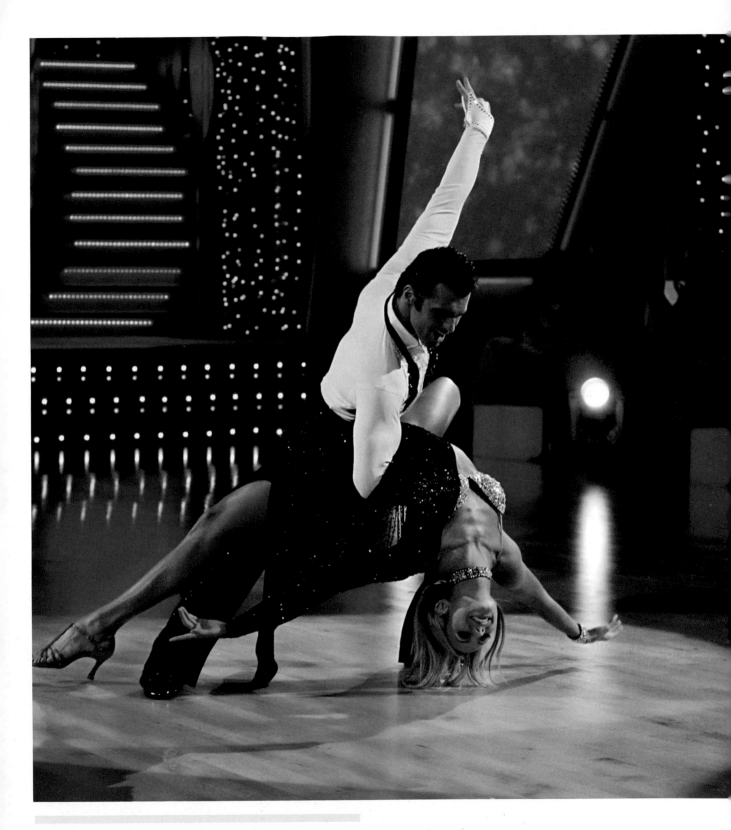

Fabulous extensions from Stacy, who manages to maintain her character despite being upside down!

samba

The ultimate party dance combines wild moves with hot Latin rhythms.

The Samba is a Brazilian party dance that can be traced back to dances brought to the New World by slaves from Africa. Samba is a Bantu word that means "pray," and the dance was used to invoke the gods. So the moves and steps were wild and lively, perfect for the numerous carnivals and street festivals in Brazil.

In the nineteenth century, the Samba steps were modified (but not compromised), and it became a partner dance.

By the 1920s, Samba gained popularity in the US, first seen in a Broadway play called *Street Carnival;* it was then made even more popular through the movies of Fred Astaire and, later, Carmen Miranda.

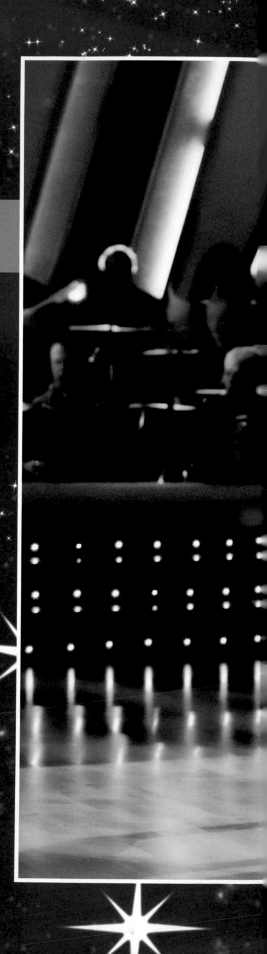

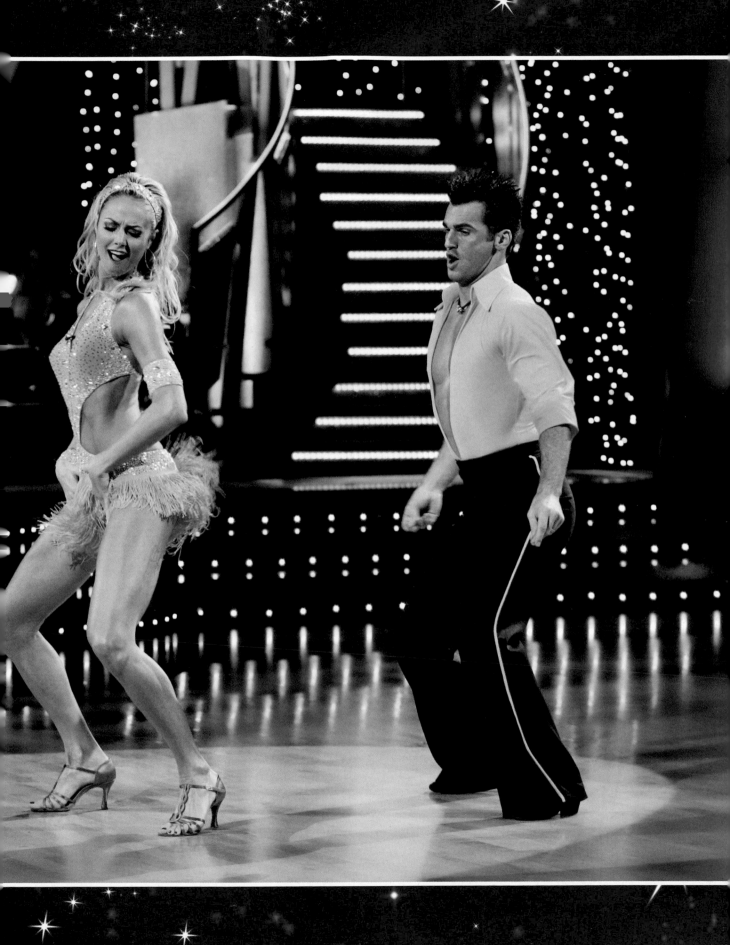

samba
a sizzling samba
Stacy Keibler and Tony Dovolani (Season 2, show 5)

Having tied for second on the leaderboard in the previous week, Stacy and Tony were determined to snatch that number one spot on Samba night.

Until now, the couple had tackled only slower dances, and so it was time for Stacy to break out of the serene and elegant mold and show her wilder side. This proved to be particularly challenging, especially when it came down to perfecting the signature hip and butt movements.

"We did four slow dances before I ever got to do a fast dance, and I was just waiting to do the Samba and the Cha-cha and shake my booty. And when we got the song "Bootylicious," we were just laughing—we were so excited to use the music. And I practiced hard. I loved it. I think that doing a dance that you like, you show your personality and it's fun, and I think that's why I got a 30—I just went out there and I let it all go. I got a 10 from Carrie Ann, I got a 10 from Len, and my heart was just beating—I didn't know what was going to happen. And then when Bruno held up that 10 I was just ecstatic. It was just such a happy moment and something that we worked really hard for."

—Stacy Keibler talking about her Samba

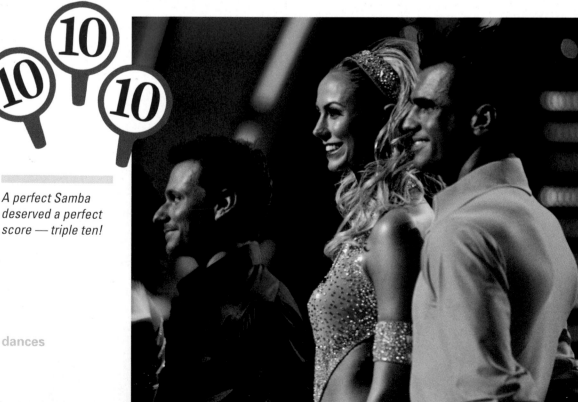

A perfect Samba deserved a perfect score — triple ten!

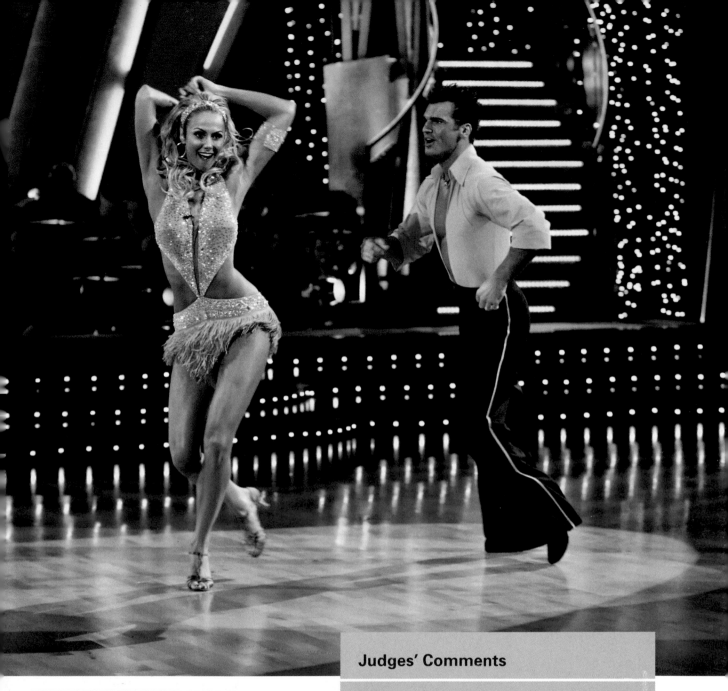

Finally given the chance to break free from the slower dances, Stacy Keibler and Tony Dovolani gave an unforgettable performance with their Samba.

However, with Tony's help and brilliant choreography, a perfect song choice, and even a visit to a Latin dance club, Stacy was able to grasp the Samba spirit and wow the judges.

Judges' Comments

Len Goodman: *"It was saucy, it was sexy, it was superb!"*

Bruno Tonioli: *"You are a weapon of mass seduction!"*

Carrie Ann Inaba: *"You are getting better than some of our professional dancers."*

samba
the look

Jerry used the vibrant carnival dance to his advantage in one of the most entertaining performances of season three. After having moved but not necessarily impressed the judges with his Waltz the week before, he made up for his lack of technique by really having fun with the Samba.

"It was the Brazil nut and the showgirl. Insanity at the Copacabana!"
—Bruno Tonioli

Since Samba is a Carnaval dance originating in Brazil, Jerry wanted them to look like a couple dancing in a parade in Brazil during Carnaval. So with that inspiration, the designers came up with Kym wearing a completely beaded gold costume, with tail feathers out of ostrich boas. Tail feathers were added on show day and carefully adjusted to stand out a bit 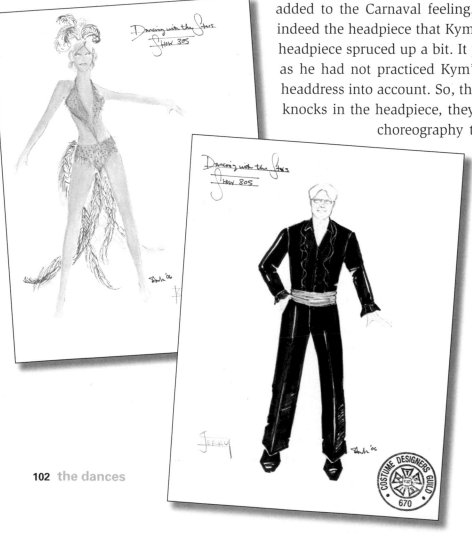 more. The pink, orange, and yellow tail-feather boas really added to the Carnaval feeling. The crowning element was indeed the headpiece that Kym wore—an original Las Vegas headpiece spruced up a bit. It presented challenges to Jerry, as he had not practiced Kym's underarm turns taking the headdress into account. So, the day of the show, after a few knocks in the headpiece, they were able to work out their choreography to incorporate the headpiece.

Kym had challenges even keeping the headpiece on, as it was a bit top heavy and was prone to flying off. After a couple of extra pieces of nude-color elastic and lots of hairpins, it was secure. The costume had to have that headdress, and Kym was a real pro to work around it.

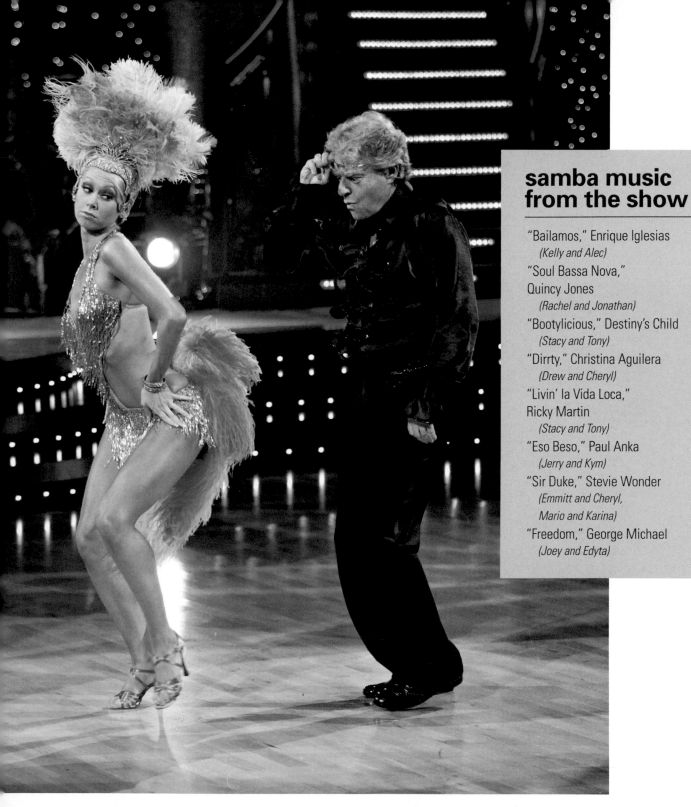

samba music
from the show

"Bailamos," Enrique Iglesias
  (Kelly and Alec)
"Soul Bassa Nova,"
Quincy Jones
  (Rachel and Jonathan)
"Bootylicious," Destiny's Child
  (Stacy and Tony)
"Dirrty," Christina Aguilera
  (Drew and Cheryl)
"Livin' la Vida Loca,"
Ricky Martin
  (Stacy and Tony)
"Eso Beso," Paul Anka
  (Jerry and Kym)
"Sir Duke," Stevie Wonder
  (Emmitt and Cheryl,
  Mario and Karina)
"Freedom," George Michael
  (Joey and Edyta)

Kym's hair was pulled into a beautiful showgirl feathery headband with bright, fun colors. Her body and face were golden and shimmery, and her eyes were layered with lashes.

Jerry Springer and Kym Johnson evoking the Carnaval, with Jerry turning the entertainment up to ten!

samba

louis van amstel's how to

- Originating from Brazil and strongly influenced by African dance, the bounce in Samba reflects the Afro-Brazilian mix.

- The Samba is the party dance, a celebration of life, like the carnival that takes place each year before Ash Wednesday. Having been to Rio De Janeiro for Carnaval, I realized the meaning of party time. Beautiful people in stunning costumes dancing until they drop!

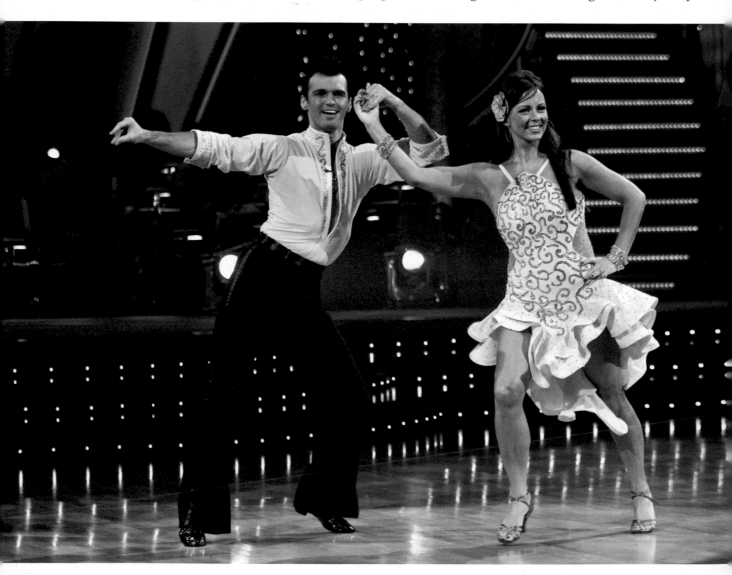

A great execution of the Promenade Botafogo. Sara and Tony show the essential Samba bounce, where the standing leg bends down into the floor, while keeping the upright posture.

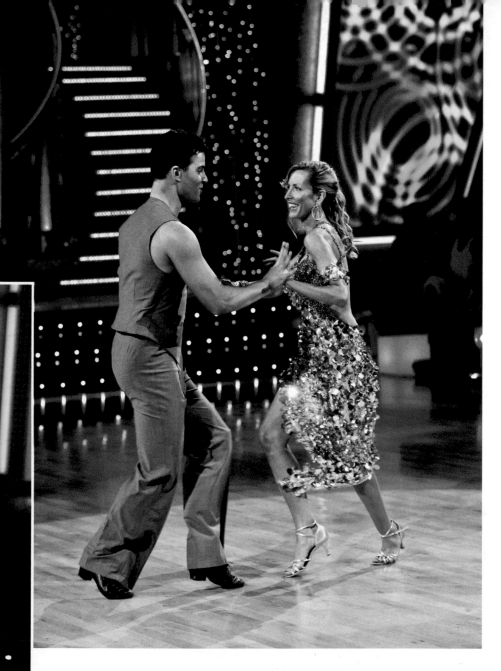

Another great example of a basic Samba figure is the Samba Locks. Heather Mills always impressed with her technique and ability to get into character for each dance. This picture shows great turnout of the feet and a very good connection within their frame.

◆ Most of the Samba has bouncy timing and is based on poly rhythms.

◆ Like the Paso Doble, the Samba has stationary and traveling figures that move anti-clockwise. Arms should be extended to achieve the correct lines.

◆ Like Cha-cha, the Samba moves forward over the ball of the foot

◆ The hips like to move in a horizontal figure of eight, with straight legs accentuating the rhythm.

samba
louis van amstel's how to

◆ The dancers want to have fun with each other due to the Samba's carnival heritage. The man does the leading, with the woman very much on show.

◆ The bounce in basic Samba has a different timing to the feet, which makes it hard to learn at first, but once mastered it gives the dancers a very grounded and earthy Samba, with fast and strong foot movement.

The party Samba, with Emmitt's sense of fun shining through. The performance was a joy to watch, and made you want to jump up and join in!

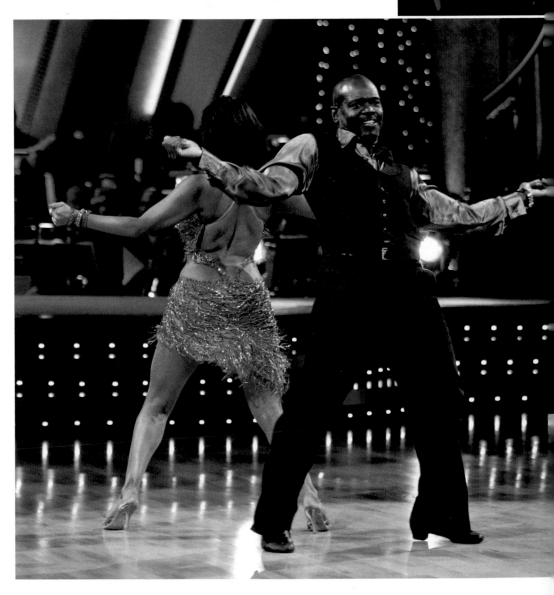

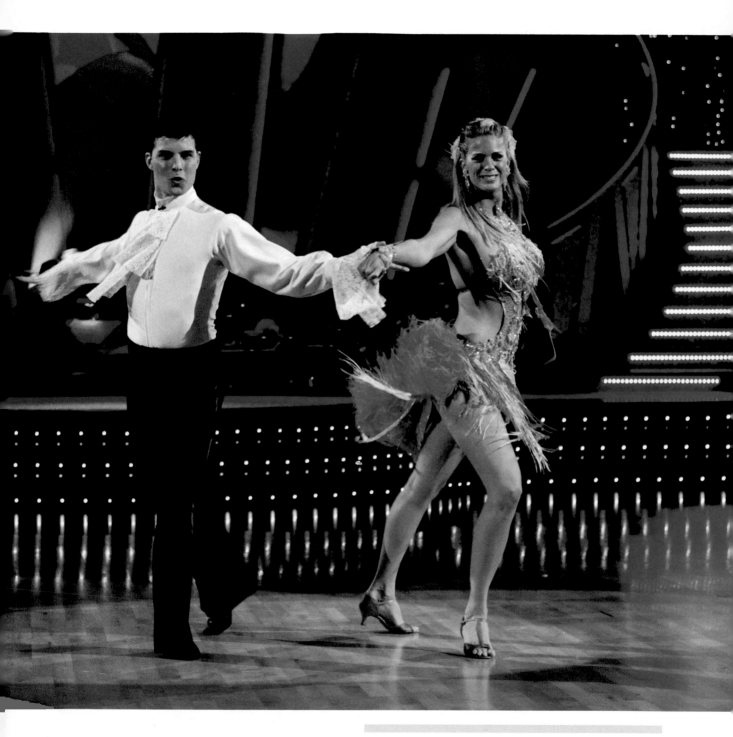

Dancers (including the celebrity dancers) use castor oil on the bottom of their dance shoes before they perform so they don't slip around too much! And sometimes the men use Vaseline on the sides of their patent leather shoes so they do slide across the floor.

Rachel Hunter and Jonathan Roberts were given a difficult piece of music for their Samba, but did brilliantly with their choreography to overcome the slowness of the piece. They created lots of bounce, and this picture shows the perfect back leg extension.

tango

The Tango is a passionate Latin dance that, when performed with the control and power it demands, can stir up real excitement.

A very controlled yet very sexy dance, the Tango originated in the poor areas of Argentina in the 1890s.

It supposedly tells the story of the gaucho and the local girl. After a day on the range, the gaucho would head to a nightclub, still in his leather chaps, which caused him to walk with flexed knees. He was also smelly from the long day, which was why the girl would dance in the crook of the gaucho's right arm, holding her head back. Her hand would rest low on his left hip, suggesting she was trying to fish for payment for the dance.

The Tango spread to Europe in the early twentieth century and was made a true hit in the US by the movie star Rudolph Valentino.

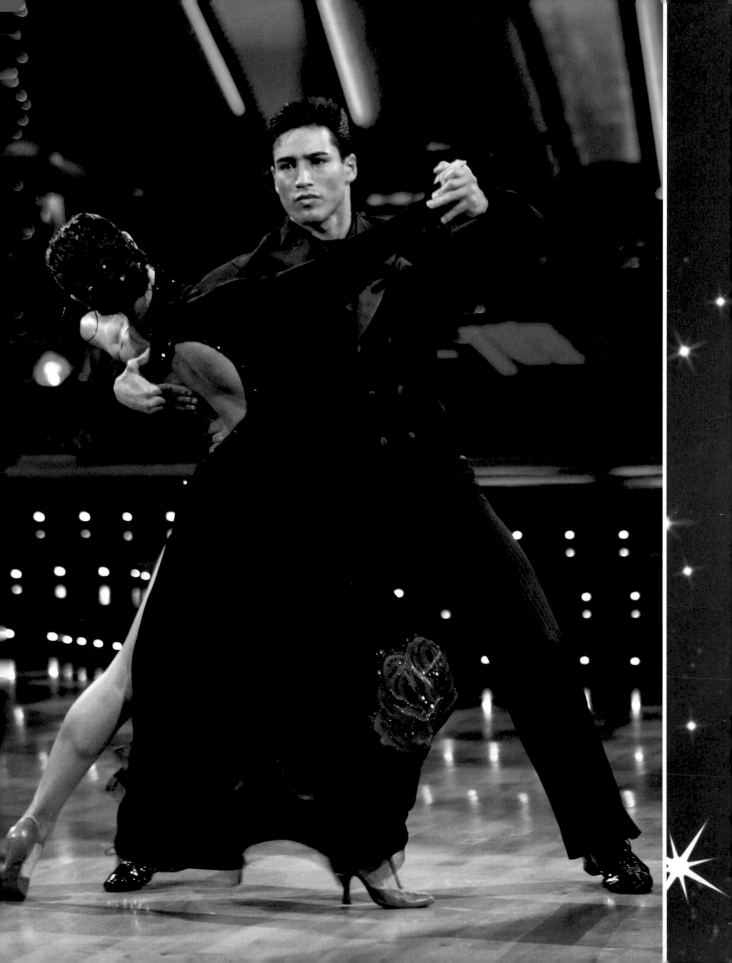

tango

a terrific tango
Mario Lopez and Karina Smirnoff (Season 3, show 3)

Mario's fiery Latin temperament combined with the passion of the Tango made this performance the most memorable (but not the best) in its category.

The week before, the couple had been reprimanded by the judges for breaking the rules in the Quickstep. So their mission was to perform the Tango by the book, without forgoing any originality.

Sparks flew on the dance floor, and although the Judges criticized their technique there was no hiding the passion.

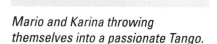

Mario and Karina throwing themselves into a passionate Tango.

However, Mario and Karina battled in rehearsal and seemingly made the wrong decisions.

"The Tango tells a love/hate story . . . like our relationship."
—Mario Lopez

Although electrifying and unique, the dance was not altogether correct and the pair were once again penalized for not following the rules.

Mario looking sheepish as Karina stands defiant in front of the Judges.

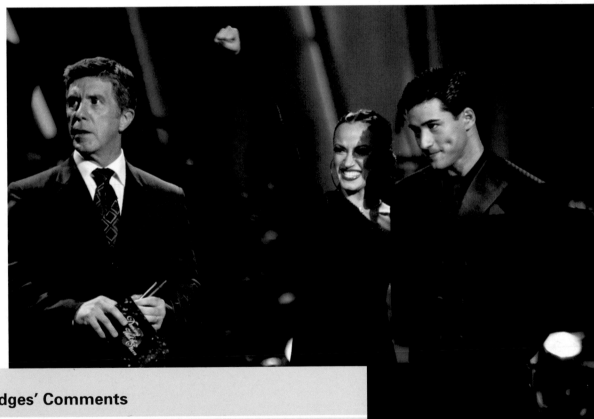

Judges' Comments

Len Goodman: *"You're off your head! I would have given you a 10. Once you broke the hold, you finished for me."*

Bruno Tonioli: *"You're a naughty boy! Why are you breaking the rules?"*

tango

the look

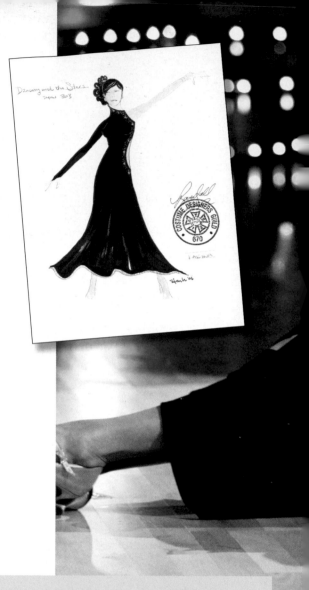

Karina had wanted to use a type of velvet that she had seen in New York: a velvet Lycra that featured a big solitary rose. The designers searched for the fabric all over downtown Los Angeles, but because that they only had two days to purchase all of the fabrics, it just didn't happen. Ultimately they found a jersey with a big, splashy red rose on it. They over-dyed it to tone down the redness of the rose, then cut it out and appliqued it onto the black velvet.

Mario wore a long line vest with satin lapels and a black shirt with black satin tie. The fabric was a black on black stripe. A red pocket square tied into Karina's red rose on her skirt. The designers tried a longer line vest but ended up drastically shortening the vest, to a drop-waist vest.

Tango looks are designed and inspired to accent the serious, passionate, and dramatic expressions of the face. Tia's look had a traditional Argentinian feel. Her hair was done up in a pulled-back side bun with a red hair tie with a sweeping side wave to accent her cheek and make-up. For the makeup, a classic red matte lip and black, smoky eye were used.

tango music from the show

"Toxic," Britney Spears
(Rachel and Jonathan)

"One Way or Another," Blondie
(Jerry and Anna)

"Shut Up," Black Eyed Peas
(Drew and Cheryl)

"Hernando's Hideaway,"
Ella Fitzgerald
(Jerry and Kym)

"Simply Irresistible,"
Robert Palmer
(Emmitt and Cheryl)

"What Are You Waiting For,"
Gwen Stefani
(Mario and Karina)

"Por Una Cabeza,"
The Tango Project
(Tia and Maksim)

"La Cumparsita,"
Danny Malando
(George and Edyta)

"Cell Block Tango,"
Chicago Soundtrack
(Stacy and Tony)

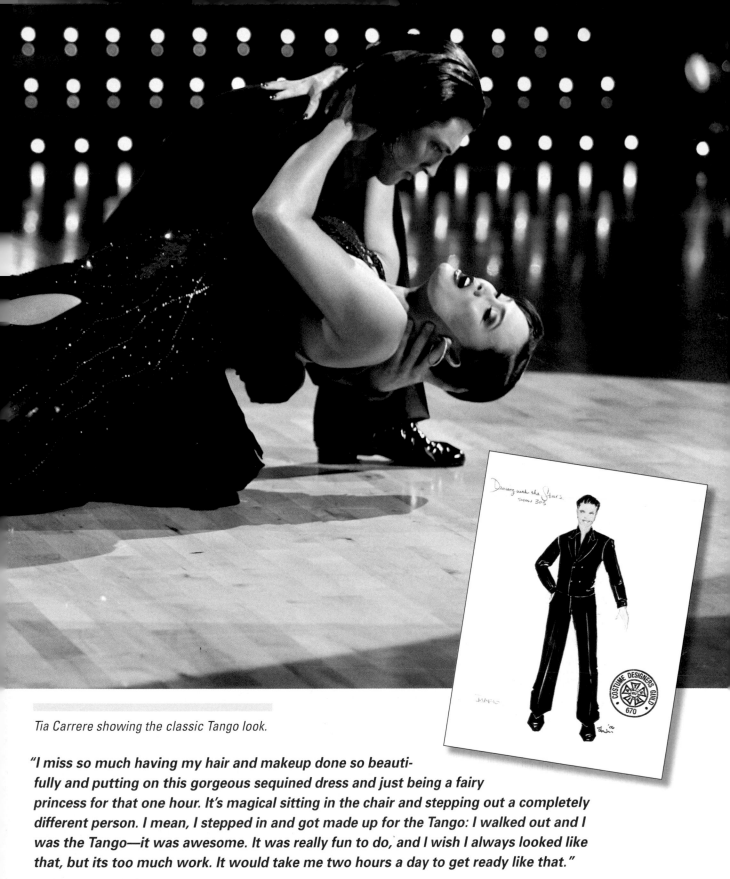

Tia Carrere showing the classic Tango look.

"*I miss so much having my hair and makeup done so beautifully and putting on this gorgeous sequined dress and just being a fairy
princess for that one hour. It's magical sitting in the chair and stepping out a completely
different person. I mean, I stepped in and got made up for the Tango: I walked out and I
was the Tango—it was awesome. It was really fun to do, and I wish I always looked like
that, but its too much work. It would take me two hours a day to get ready like that.*"

—Tia Carrere, talking about her hair, makeup and wardrobe

louis van amstel's how to

◆ The Tango is the most passionate and aggressive of the ballroom dances and is totally distinct from the others. While the other ballroom dances want to be smooth and full of swing, the Tango has no swing at all.

◆ The Tango has no rise and fall, with lots of staccato movement exchanged with some legato (slow) movement, which gives the dancers the opportunity to be very powerful and yet remain calm. The knees remain slightly bent throughout, and great control is needed to perfect the stalking style of the Tango.

◆ Like the Quickstep, the Tango is performed in the international style, which means the same rules apply.

The great entertainer George Hamilton here captures the Argentinian flavor of the Tango.

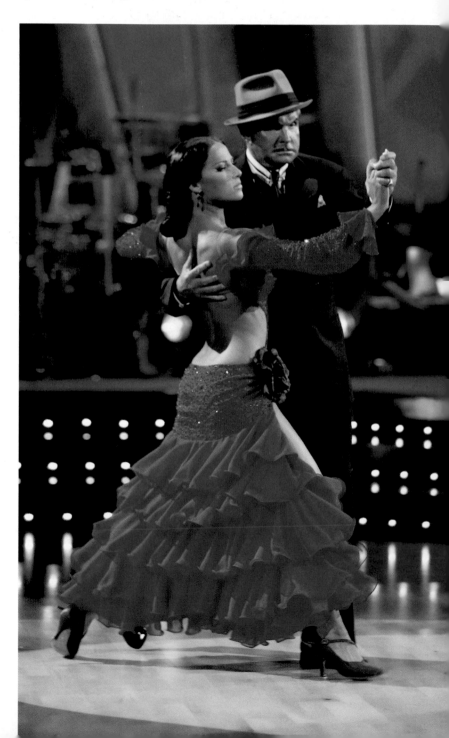

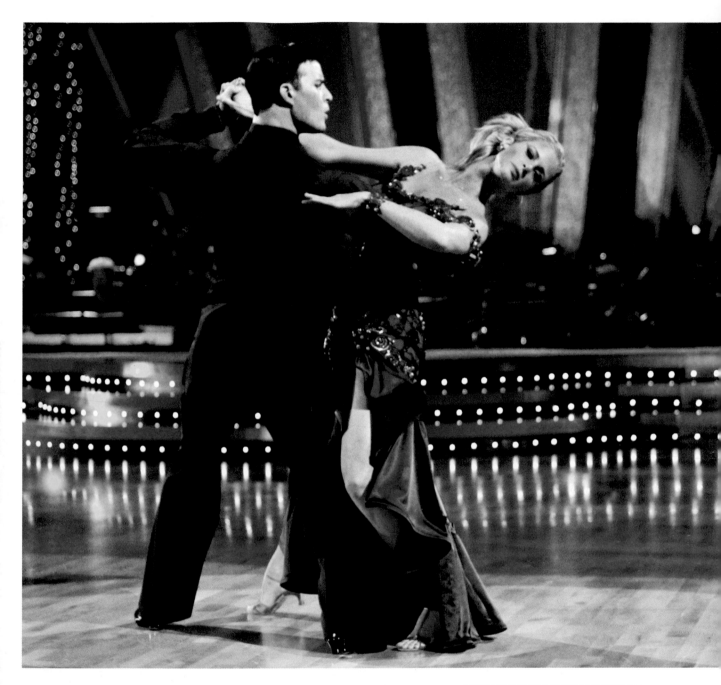

While the American-style Foxtrot and Waltz allow the dancers to be open and don't require close holds, leaving the dancers more vulnerable, the Tango is even more difficult because of the risk of tripping over each others feet and maintaining the correct posture. The arms are not so outstretched, and the dancers hold is close, allowing the man to whisk the woman into dramatic positions.

It's very difficult to keep an open posture in the close hold, but Rachel here does a beautiful job, staying as open as possible despite the heat of the dance.

tango

louis van amstel's how to

◆ All forward steps are taken on the heel; legs are always bent; and there is lots of tension between the partners. The Argentinian heritage of the Tango often gives the tension and erotic edge.

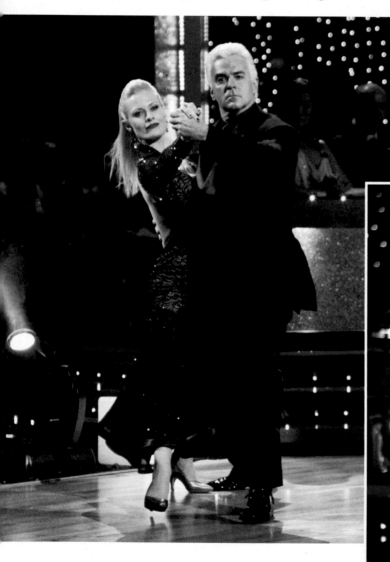

A great example of an inner calmness, and yet with fire in the eyes. John's posture and footwork were probably his greatest assets during season one.

In regular competition a close hold must be maintained, but on the show there is a little more freedom. Harry Hamlin and Ashly here have also chosen an Argentinian flavor, but keeping the close hold and portraying a passionate intensity.

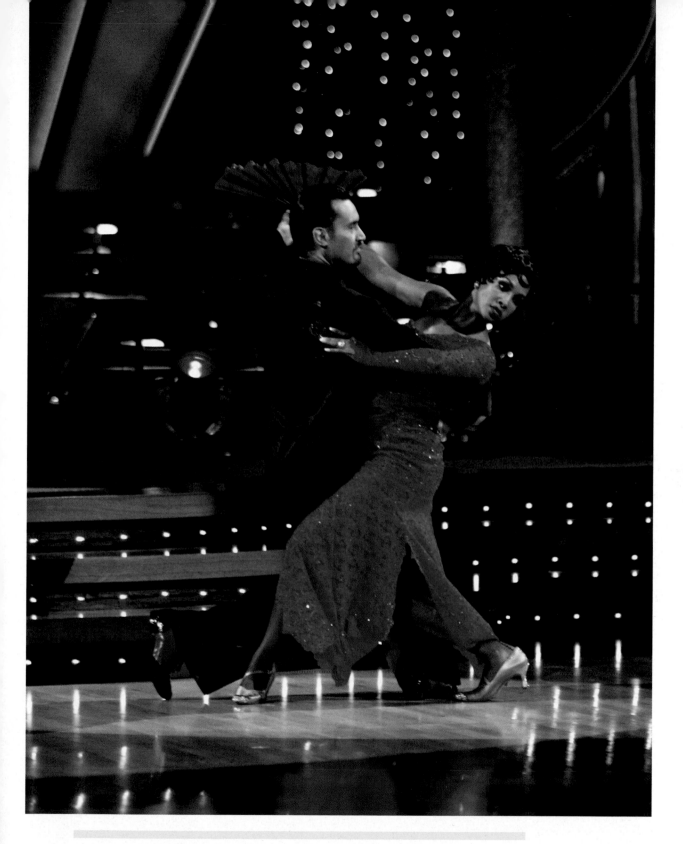

Vivica and Nick showing the perfect international-style Tango hold, while presenting a beautiful Contra-Check. You can also see that there is absolutely no space between Vivica and Nick's mid-torso and hips, a very difficult thing to achieve.

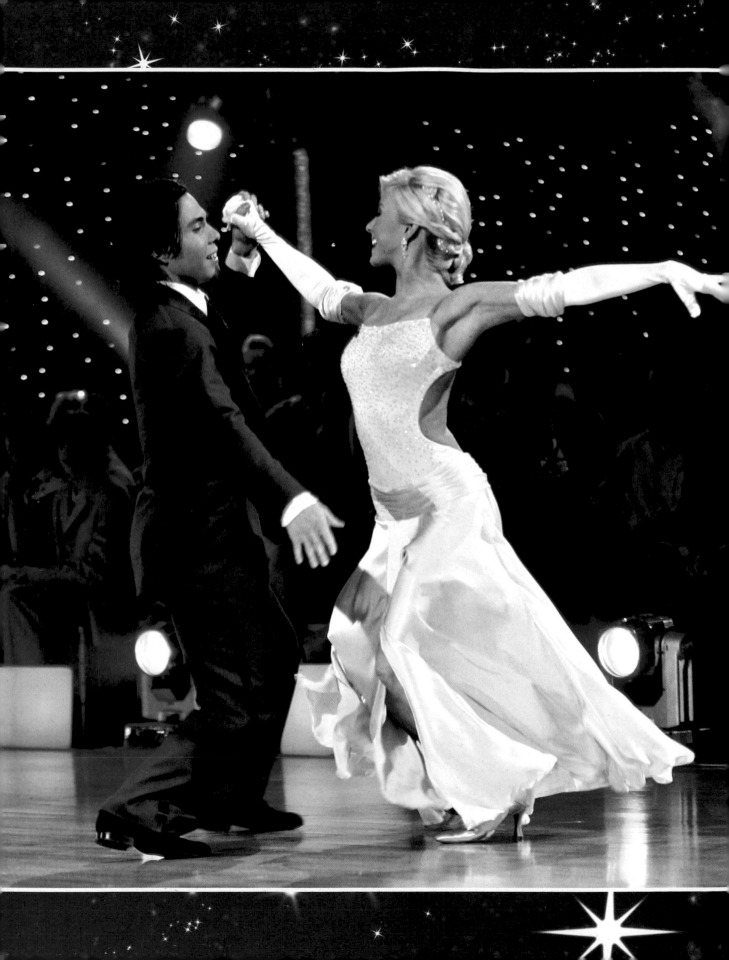

waltz

The most elegant and traditional of ballroom dances, it relies on total communication between the couple or it can be disastrous!

Although now regarded as one of the most old-fashioned and elegant forms of ballroom dancing, the Waltz was once seen as incredibly scandalous.

It was originally a French peasant dance and became popular in Vienna, Austria, in the eighteenth century. When it was introduced in England and the US, however, it was criticized heavily for its sexual overtones; men and women were closely intertwined. Nevertheless, this distaste only encouraged curiosity and eventually the dance caught on.

waltz

a wonderful waltz
Apolo Anton Ohno and Julianne Hough (Season 4, show 4)

Dancing greatness often begins with a great couple, and from the start Apolo and Julianne were a perfect match. Their Waltz divided the judges, drawing glowing praise from Carrie Ann and Bruno for their style and romance and yet criticism from Len for lack of technique. What is certain is that the audience loved the performance and really took the couple to their hearts. Apolo and Julianne were able to take the competition to a new level and set the bar higher for the other stars who followed.

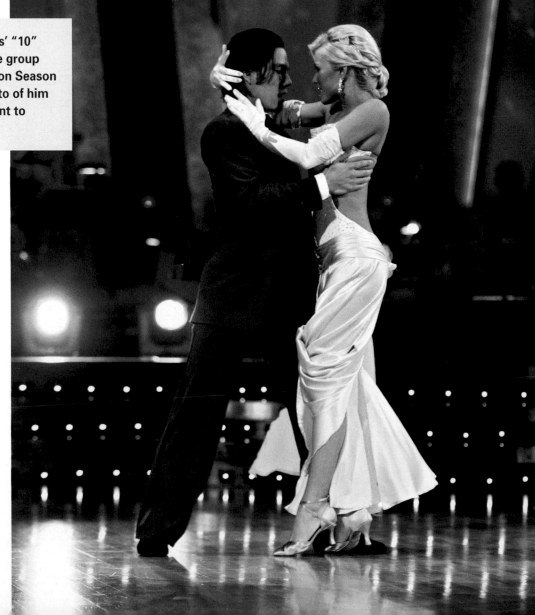

Ian stole a Judges' "10" paddle during the group Swing rehearsal on Season 4 and took a photo of him with it that he sent to Joey & Apolo!

The winners of Season 4 beginning to show their strength. Apolo and Julianne deliver a faultless Waltz.

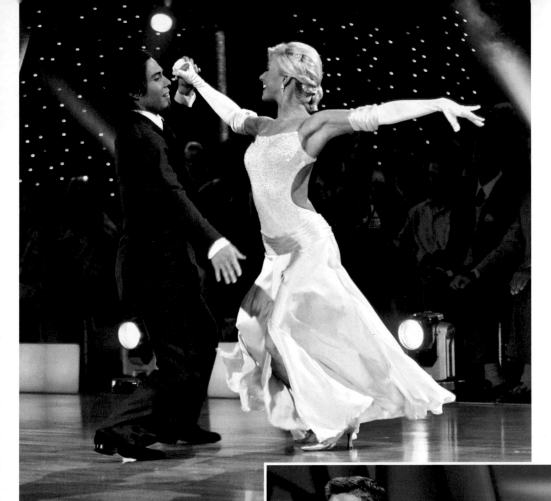

A fantastic couple, who complemented and inspired each other perfectly.

Judges' Comments

Carrie Ann Inaba: *"Yeah! I believed every minute of it. That was so romantic, that was wonderful."*

Bruno Tonioli: *"The dream team—it's like finally I'm seeing the crown jewels of the competition . . . . You gave a lovely story. I believed the romance."*

Len Goodman: *"Learning a routine is not the end of it: that's the start of it."*

High praise from the Judges.

waltz
the look

Stacy's first costume was one of the designers' all-time favorites. To come out on the very first show in such an incredible gown had to have taken quite a bit of courage. Stacy's costume consisted of criss-cross ruching over the bust, one side black, one side fuchsia, wrapping around the small of her back and attaching to the drop-waist skirt. The high slit in the skirt really showed off her legs and her fabulous extensions! Her first kick blew everyone away. Such grace on such a tall and statuesque beauty.

Both Stacy and Willa had classic looks, with soft sophisticated makeup and hair details, with elegant up-do's to show the lines of the arms and shoulders. For Willa a black, rhinestone, smoky eye with a nude lip added a little drama.

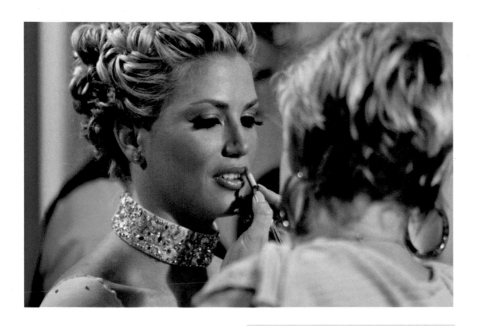

Head of makeup Melanie Mills applies the finishing touches to Willa Ford.

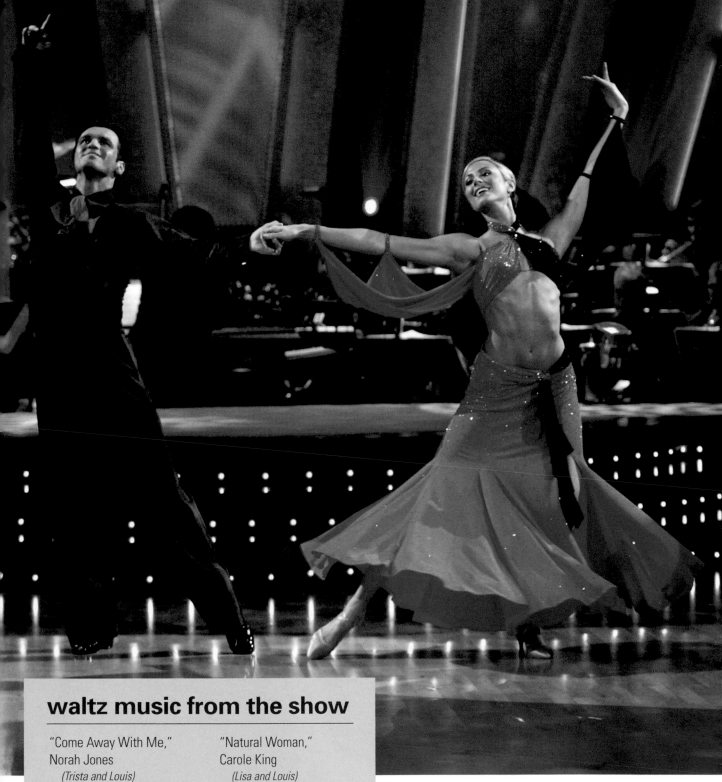

waltz music from the show

"Come Away With Me,"
Norah Jones
　(Trista and Louis)

"Three Times A Lady,"
The Commodores
　(Rachel and Jonathan)

"What A Wonderful World,"
Ross Mitchell
　(Tia and Maksim)

"Natural Woman,"
Carole King
　(Lisa and Louis)

"Take It To The Limit,"
The Eagles
　(Joey and Edyta)

"Tennessee Waltz,"
Patti Page
　(Jerry and Kym)

Stacy Keibler in her spectacular Waltz costume. A great costume can really add another dimension to a performance.

waltz
louis van amstel's how to

◆ Unlike other ballroom dances on the show, the Waltz is performed to a three-quarter beat, which can be quite a hurdle to learn at first, since we are used to a four-four beat.

◆ Because of the swing in this dance, the couple has the opportunity to create beautiful rises and falls without any sudden or direct interruptions.

◆ Symmetry plays a key part, with the partners' legs often mirroring each other. The basic hold remains solid throughout.

◆ This dance is considered the most sensitive or spiritual dance in ballroom, and therefore gives the opportunity to show off beautiful lines and movement and to be the most expressive.

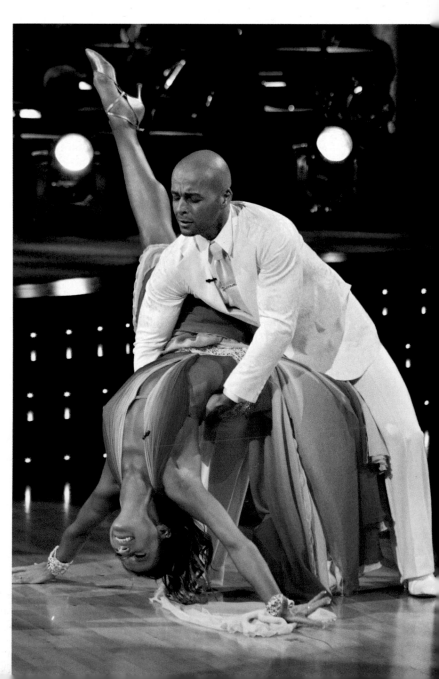

A perfect example of why the American-style ballroom creates opportunities to dazzle. This gorgeous line created by Joey Lawrence and Edyta was typical of the excellence they brought to the Waltz.

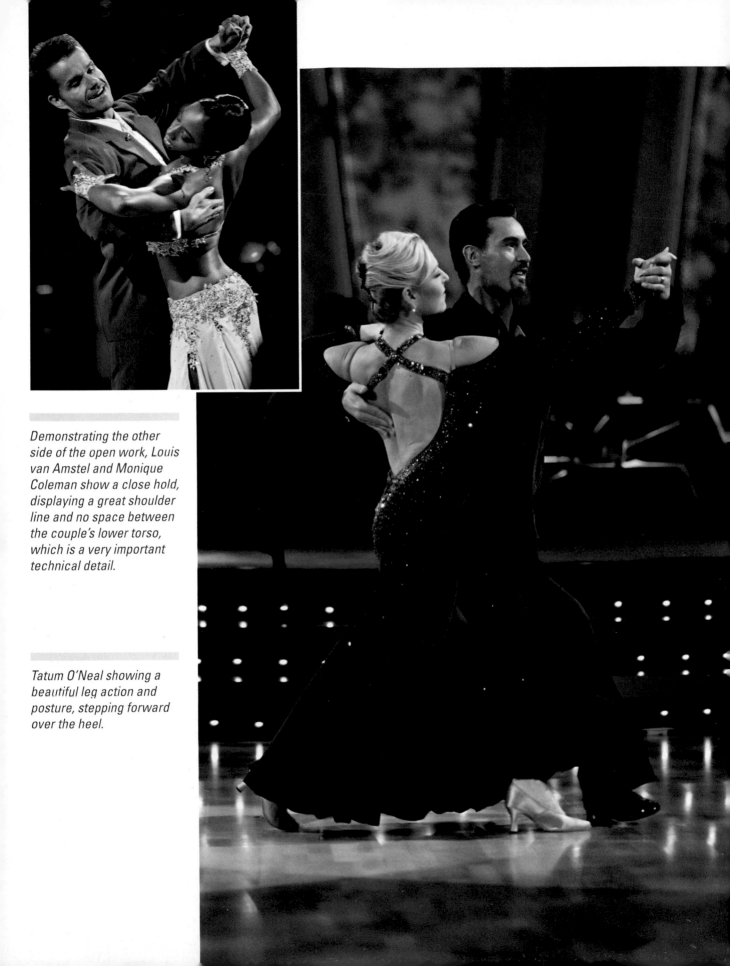

Demonstrating the other side of the open work, Louis van Amstel and Monique Coleman show a close hold, displaying a great shoulder line and no space between the couple's lower torso, which is a very important technical detail.

Tatum O'Neal showing a beautiful leg action and posture, stepping forward over the heel.

waltz
louis van amstel's how to

◆ Waltz steps go forward over the heel, then on the ball of the foot while rising up. Stepping and turning is in the classic one-two-three rhythm.

◆ In international competitions, where there are at least six couples competing at one time, the dancers move anti-clockwise around the floor. On *Dancing with the Stars,* there is more leniency with this rule as the couple is alone on the floor.

After all of their high-energy dancing, Mario and Karina were able to turn around and perform a calm, beautiful, and highly spiritual Waltz.

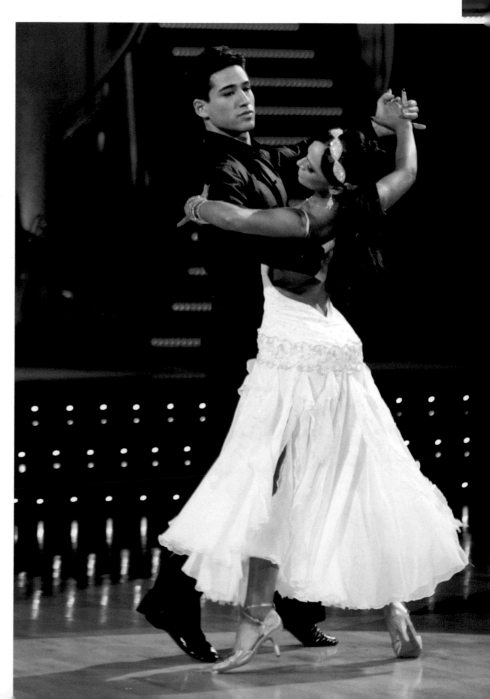

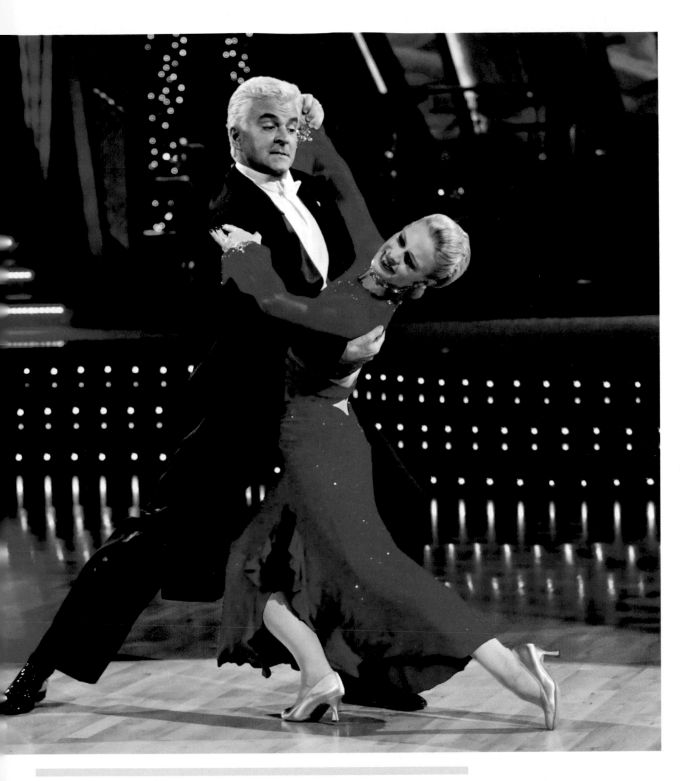

John demonstrates a perfect Throwaway Oversway and his reputation for great posture in the ballroom dances. In this line, the man dances the woman around in front of him before turning her and allowing her torso to extend back.

who could forget . . .?

In four fantastic seasons, there have been countless incredible dances, touching stories, and wonderful moments. Here are some more of the most unforgettable.

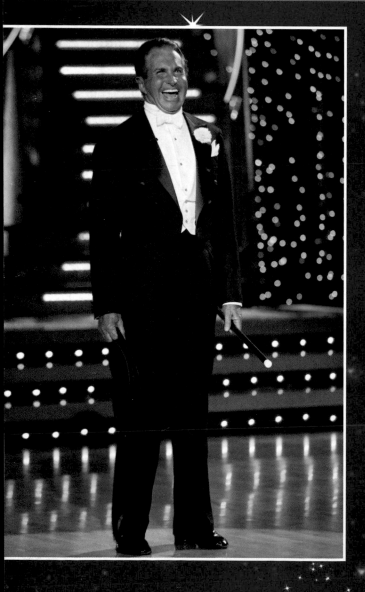

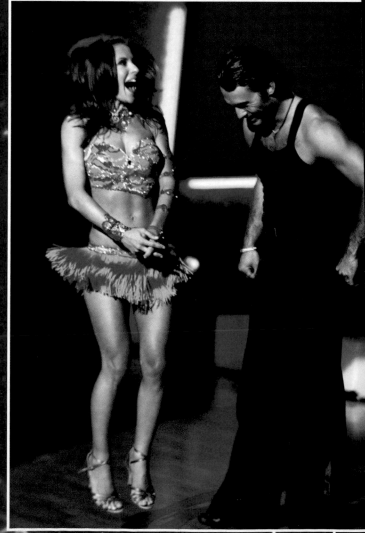

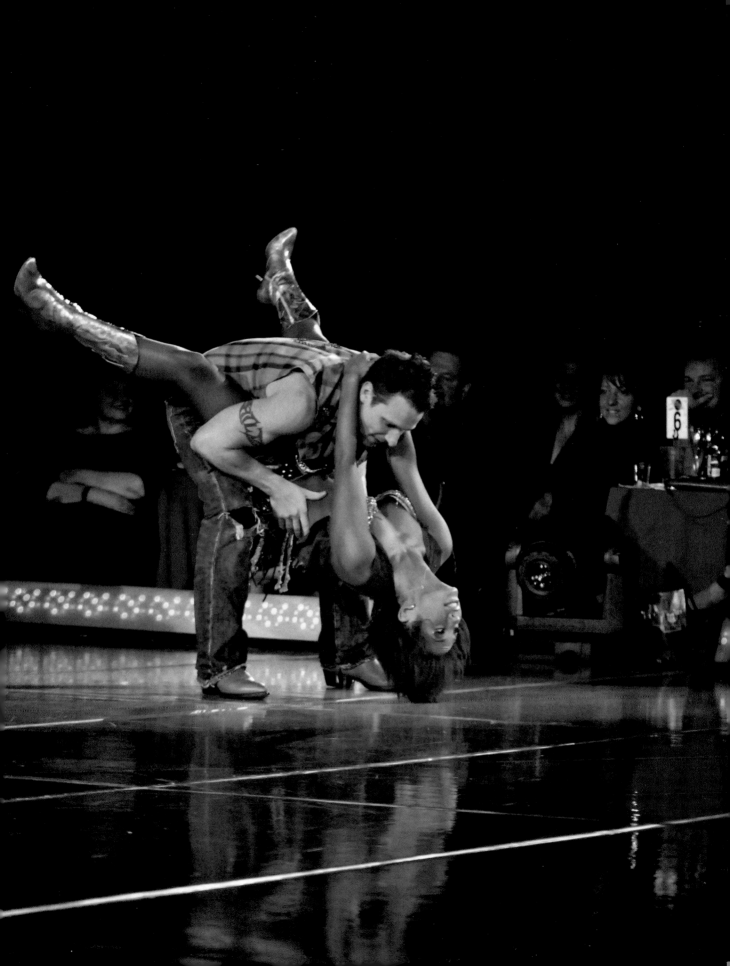

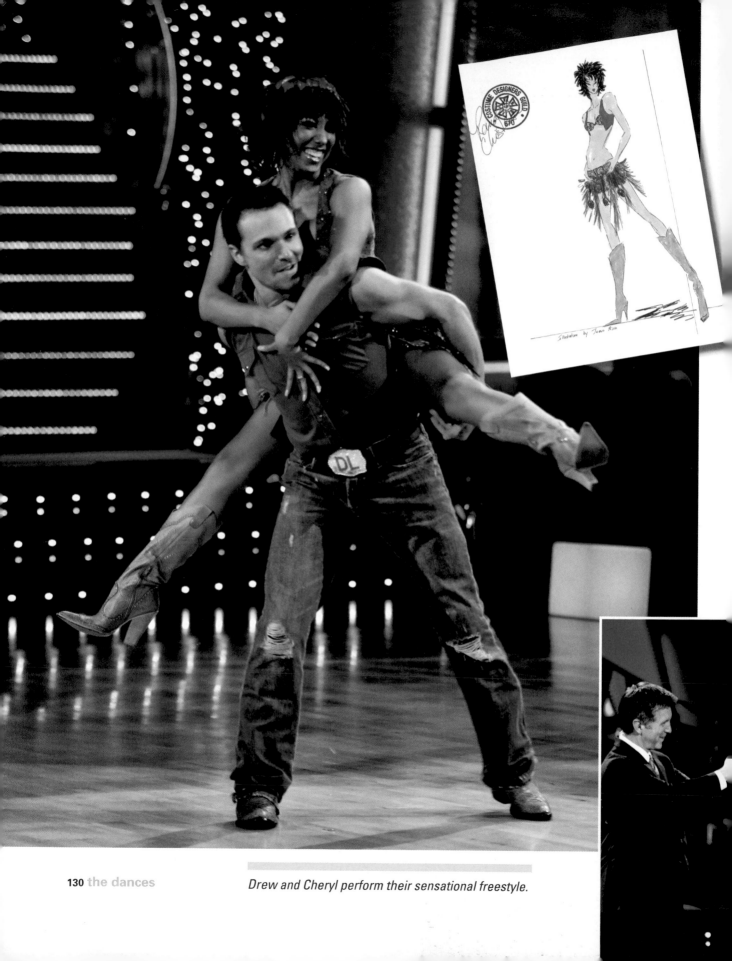

Drew and Cheryl perform their sensational freestyle.

drew and cheryl's freestyle

Season 2, show 8. "Save a Horse, Ride a Cowboy," Big and Rich.
Also seen in the *Dancing with the Stars* tour, 2006.

Drew and Cheryl pulled out all the stops for the finale with their Western-themed Freestyle dance.

Clad in sparkly cowboy attire, they dazzled the judges with their fearless moves and their unbreakable confidence, scoring a much-coveted triple 10.

"We've been living with these regulations for eight weeks now, so to have all the rules gone and to be able to get out there and do what you want to do is great. It's very liberating."

—Drew Lachey, talking about his Freestyle

This dance truly broke free of the shackles of the ballroom, with a unique Western style and choreography that lit up the dance floor. While "Thriller'" had shown how Drew and Cheryl were able to bring a contemporary feel to a ballroom dance, "Save a Horse, Ride a Cowboy" showed what they could do with no rules at all. Drew is a born showman, and from the first leap the crowd loved his athletic performance and the energy he was able to bring back time and time again when they took the dance on tour.

"Creating a costume that was both sexy and yet a 'dance' look while staying true to the Western style was a real challenge. I shopped all over Los Angeles and Beverly Hills to find just the right tassels, bellpulls,

Judges' Comments

Len Goodman: *"That was everything Freestyle should be. It was fun. You went right to the edge. It was entertaining. It was brilliant."*

Bruno Tonioli: *"Drew, you are ready for the lead role in* Brokeback Mountain, the Musical! *You're a star!"*

Carrie Ann Inaba: *"It was exciting; it was powerful; it was passionate. It was everything you know how to bring to the dance floor when it matters."*

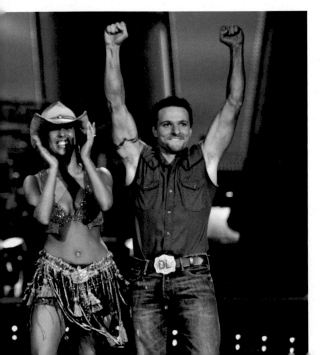

and fringing that would become her belt. I spent more time on that belt than any other costume before or since, and I knew we had a hit when everyone commented on the belt and asked where we got it. The costume was eventually auctioned off for a charity in Cheryl's hometown."

—Randall Christensen, costume designer for
Dancing with the Stars

Celebrating the Judges' comments

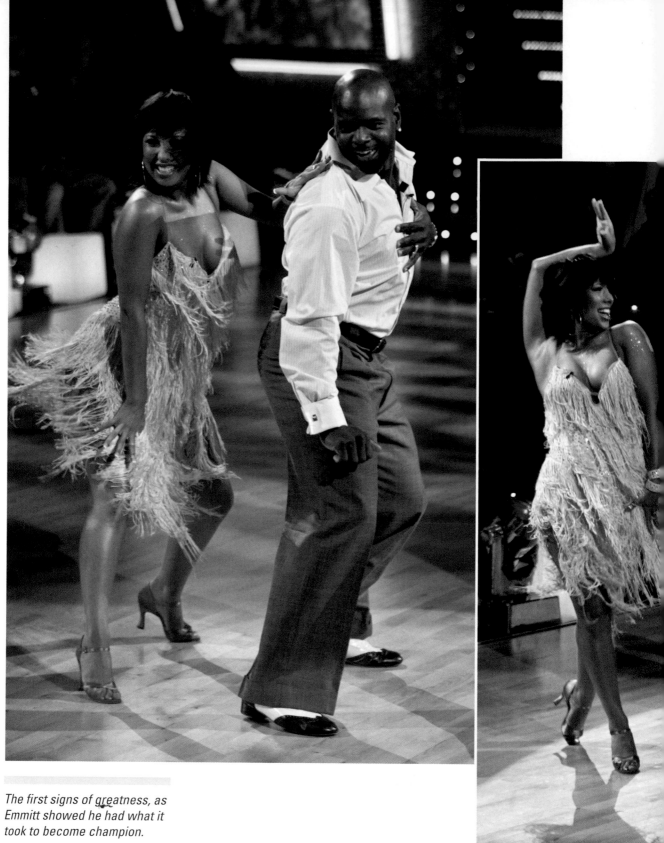

The first signs of greatness, as Emmitt showed he had what it took to become champion.

emmitt and cheryl's cha-cha

Season 3, show 1.
"Son of a Preacher Man," Dusty Springfield.

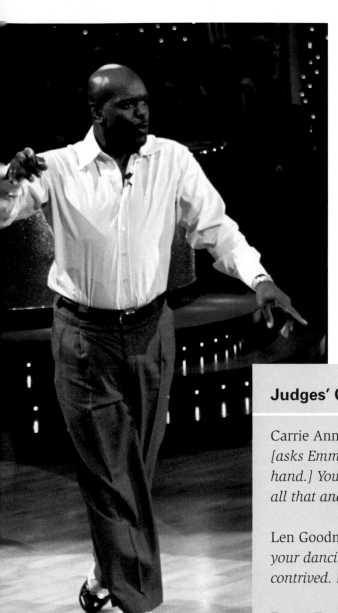

Who knew Emmitt Smith could dance?

Former NFL player Emmitt Smith surprised everybody with his very first dance of the competition, and became a breakout star overnight.

In the training leading up to the performance, his partner, Cheryl Burke, fined him fifty cents every time he led with his heels. Needless to say, he built up quite a debt that week!

Nevertheless, it was a fruitful exercise. Emmitt wowed the judges with his Cha-cha (which included a taste of the "Electric Boogaloo"), bringing Carrie Ann and the audience to a standing ovation.

Judges' Comments

Carrie Ann Inaba: *"Could you come here sir? [asks Emmitt to come over so she can shake his hand.] You can dance! That was great! You were all that and then some. Good job."*

Len Goodman: *"You've got a naturalness about your dancing, which is charming—it's not contrived. It was a joy."*

Bruno Tonioli: *"Man, you are the king of effortless cool. For the first time tonight I wanted to join in and dance."*

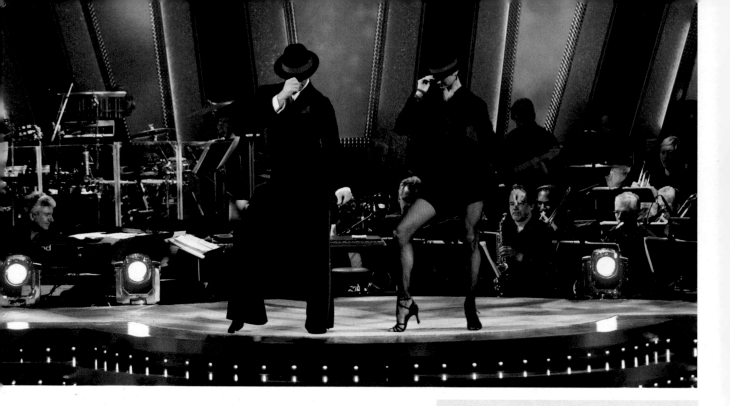

stacy and tony's jive
Season 2, show 6 & 8. "Wake Me Up Before You Go-Go," Wham!

The Jive originally caught on when American GIs brought it over to Europe during the Second World War.

So during the week leading up to her performance, Stacy Keibler decided to visit the troops at Camp Pendleton and dedicate her dance to them. While there, she acted as drill sergeant and got the troops marching and even had her dance partner, Tony Dovolani, do push-ups for the crowd.

Her patriotic spirit shone through in her performance on show night, when she gained a triple-10 score from the judges.

Judges' Comments

Bruno Tonioli: *"Well, the Jive, excitement, energy, fast pace, precise, kicks, flicks, pivot turns . . . you did them all like a bombshell! And you made it sexy as hell."*

Len Goodman: *"Well, you know, I had a feeling with your long legs, you might be like a daddy longlegs, but you weren't—your kicks were sharp. It was absolutely spot-on again, well done, Tony, well done.*

Carrie Ann Inaba: *"OK, there is nothing to say except that was pretty much perfect."*

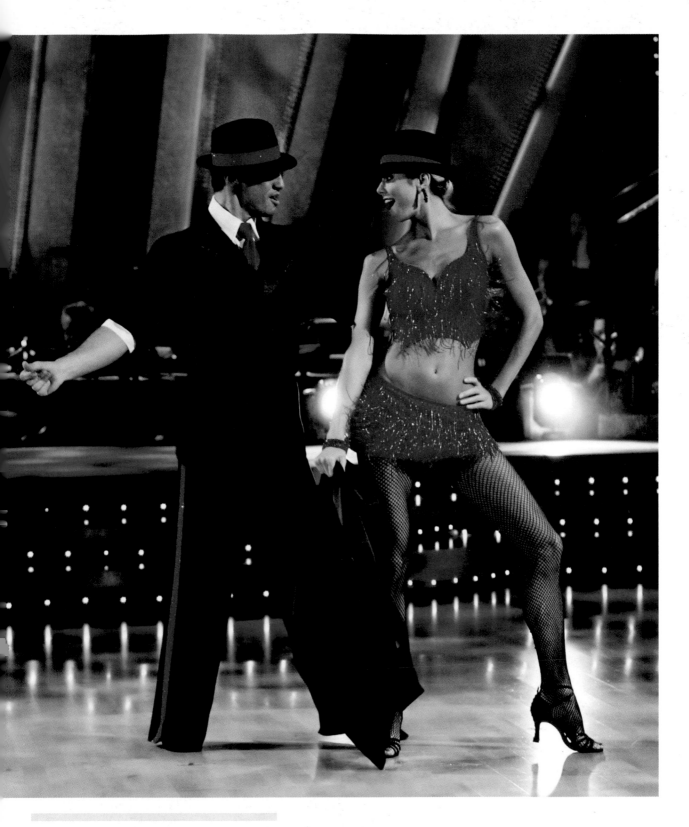

An electric performance brought the fans to their feet and had the Judges in raptures.

lisa and louis's quickstep
Season 3, show 6. "Nine to Five," Dolly Parton.

Up until this point, Lisa Rinna had truly excelled in Latin dances, but had yet to prove herself in ballroom.

So in the week before her Quickstep, she visited an etiquette teacher, who helped her adopt the elegant ballroom demeanor by balancing books on her head, and even showing her how to drink tea properly!

It seemed to do the trick, as her performance was absolutely fantastic, ending with Lisa running up the stairs above the band.

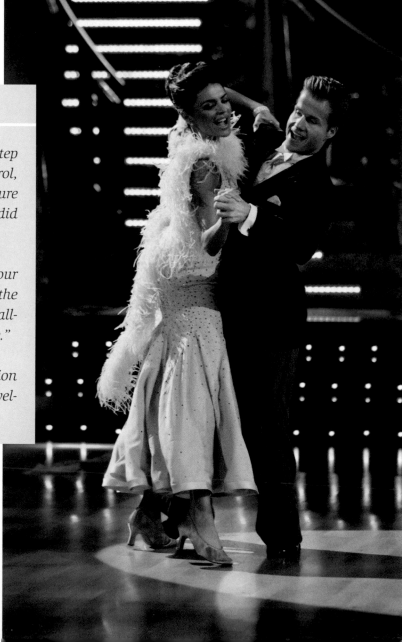

Judges' Comments

Len Goodman: *"In the Quickstep you want to see speed and control, you've got to have a lovely posture and great movement—and you did exactly that."*

Carrie Ann Inaba: *"I think that your fear of ballroom should go out of the window because you can do ballroom, girl. You had great posture."*

Bruno Tonioli: *"The emancipation of Lisa is now complete. Lisa, welcome to the ball."*

Lisa banished her ballroom fears with this sensational Quickstep.

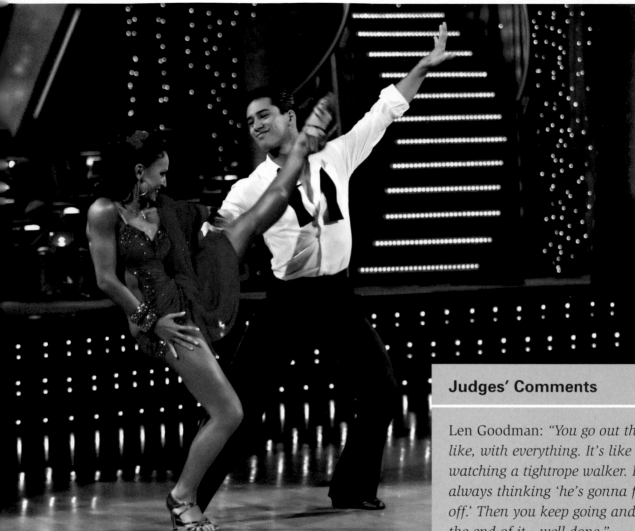

mario and karina's rumba
Season 3, show 5.
"The Way You Look Tonight," Michael Bublé.

Mario Lopez and Karina Smirnoff's romance had been much speculated about throughout the series, and it was in this performance that it really came to light.

During the previous week's training, the couple couldn't keep their hands or eyes off each other, which really helped them perfect their Rumba, otherwise known as the dance of love.

Judges' Comments

Len Goodman: *"You go out there, like, with everything. It's like watching a tightrope walker. I'm always thinking 'he's gonna fall off.' Then you keep going and at the end of it—well done."*

Bruno Tonioli: *"Well, again, intense, throbbing, steaming, and masterful. You two make such a package. I don't know what you're doing after hours, but it works on the dance floor."*

Carrie Ann Inaba: *"You're fabulous. You're fabulous."*

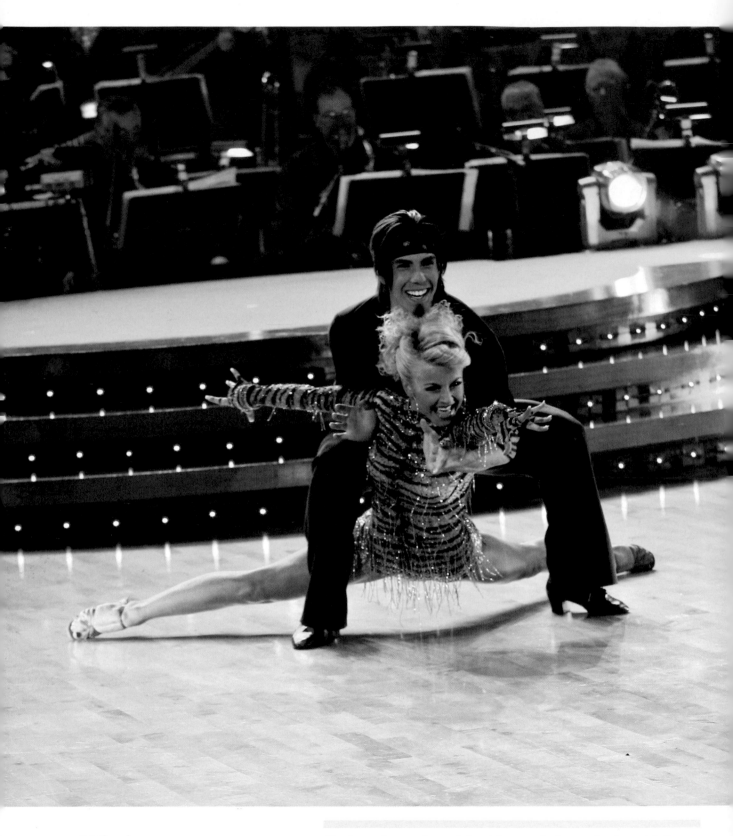

The inner tiger and a real tiger! Season 4 winners Apolo and Julianne.

apolo and julianne's samba
Season 4, show 5. "I Like to Move It," Reel 2 Real.

The Samba was Julianne Hough's favorite dance, so Apolo Anton Ohno was determined not to let her down.

By his own admission, Apolo wasn't the most fiery of dancers, so he spent training week perfecting his inner tiger!

To encourage Apolo in the actual performance, Julianne wore a tiger-print bodysuit, which clearly worked, as the couple scored the first triple 10 of the season.

Judges' Comments

Len Goodman: *"You know, occasionally the music, the choreography, the performance, all come together and you get a great, great show. That was excellent."*

Bruno Tonioli: *"You two were possessed tonight. You were like two bewitching devils on this dance floor, and I think the nation has been stunned. This is incredible!"*

Carrie Ann Inaba: *"Perfection! That's it, perfection. That was perfect!"*

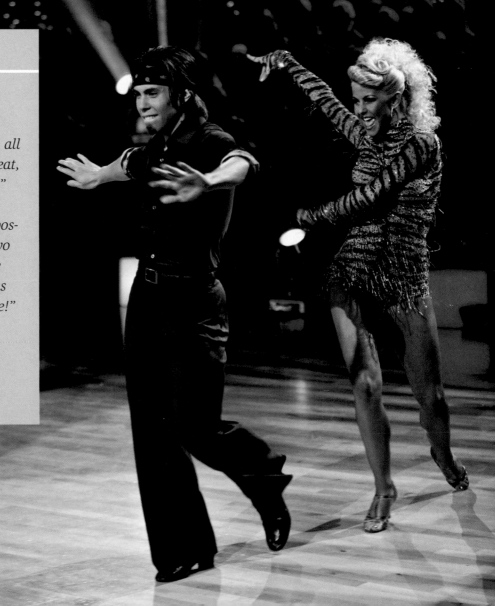

The couple brought fabulous choreography together with faultless technique.

joey and kym's tango
Season 4, show 3. *Star Wars* theme, John Williams.

This Tango was particularly memorable because of its *Star Wars* theme.

An old friend of *Star Wars* creator George Lucas, Joey got permission to use a real light saber in the performance and R2D2 in practice. He also donned an authentic Jedi braid, which was stuck to the back of his head with extra-strength glue! Kym Johnson dressed as Princess Leia, and her costume was a true hit, especially with George Lucas, who was apparently quite taken with the new Leia.

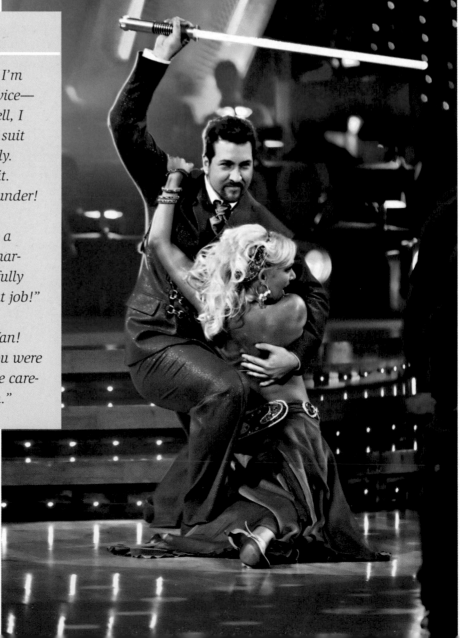

Judges' Comments

Len Goodman: *"It was good. I'm gonna give you one bit of advice—your bum sticks out a bit. Well, I know it's big, but your towel suit last week covered it over lovely. This didn't—it sticks out a bit. Get those towels on—tuck it under!"*

Carrie Ann Inaba: *"That was a well-rehearsed, tight, solid, charismatic, entertaining, beautifully performed performance. Great job!"*

Bruno Tonioli: *"Great, Obi-Wan! The Force is still with you! You were holding your spare so well. Be careful sometimes with your bum."*

Combining Joey's love of Star Wars *with Kym's fabulous choreography created an instant classic.*

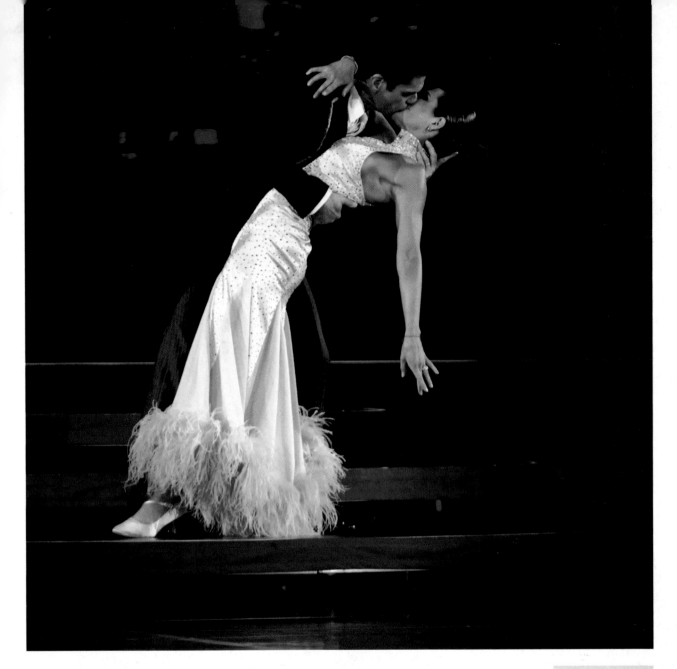

harry hamlin and wife, lisa rinna, finally getting to dance

A romantic Waltz between husband and wife.

Watching his wife Lisa compete in Season 2 inspired Harry to take to the ballroom himself in Season 3. United on the *Dancing with the Stars* tour they were finally able to dance together, choosing a romantic Waltz that took them back to their wedding day. Never before or since have two stars danced together without a professional partner.

Groundbreakers

Learning each new dance in only a week is a tough challenge, but some of the stars managed to show that they could battle all the odds.

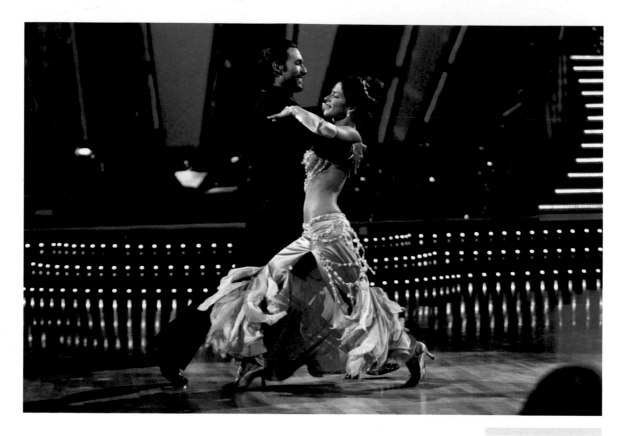

Kelly Monaco, the Underdog

Kelly's ability soared during Season 1.

Kelly Monaco's first performance on the show was met with disappointment by the judges. Carrie Ann simply did not enjoy her dancing, and Bruno Tonioli, exhibiting what was to become his trademark bluntness, asked, "Is there a death in the family?" She scored a very weak 13.

"I got creamed and it was difficult, but I chose to take a different route and better myself and better my ability and work a little harder, because that's the only way you're going to make anything in life. If you keep letting things bring you down, that's where you're going to stay. So I decided to take the higher road and put in the effort and work really hard and get through it."

—Kelly Monaco

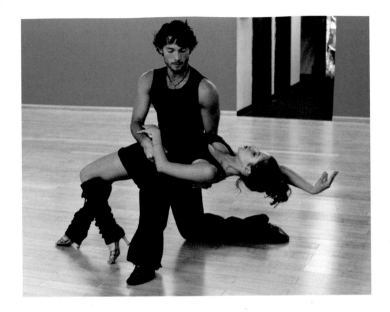

Through countless hours of hard work Kelly transformed herself into a dancer.

And work hard she did.

Despite having to juggle her training with her busy *General Hospital* schedule, and despite an embarrassing "wardrobe malfunction" in her first Samba in show four, Kelly made incredible strides.

Every week her scores escalated and she remained in the competition through the finale, in which she stunned the judges with her final Freestyle dance.

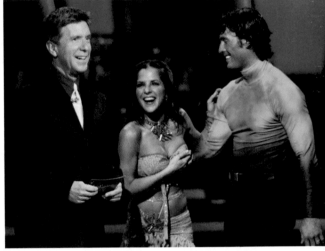

The practice starts to pay off.

Not only did Kelly get the first 10 of the series; she got the perfect triple 10 and was crowned the winner of season one.

A fairytale ending: Kelly and Alec won the first season.

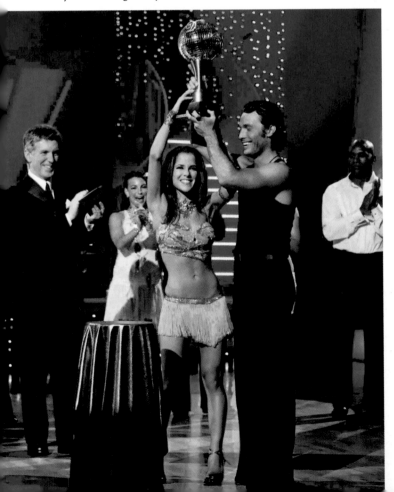

Judges' Comments

Len Goodman: *"That was unbelievably great . . . the performance of the whole series."*

Carrie Ann Inaba: *"Are you that same girl I called an awkward mover?"*

Bruno Tonioli: *"Hot hot hot hot."*

Tia Carrere, the Transformation

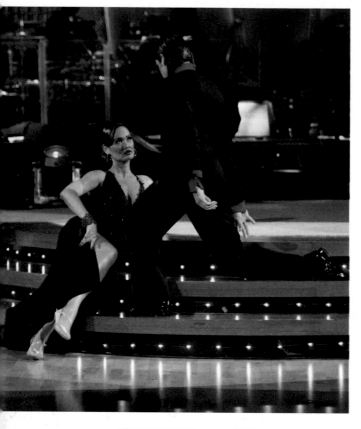

Tia smolders once again.

When Tia Carrere was invited to appear on *Dancing with the Stars,* she had her reservations. Having given birth only a few weeks earlier, she had experienced some weight gain and wasn't the Tia Carrere we all knew from *Wayne's World* and *True Lies.*

"It was scary as an actress to appear on television heavier than I had ever been in my life. Many women were saying, 'It's so brave of you to go out there,' and I think they meant, 'It's so brave of you to go out there as big as you are right now!'"
—Tia Carrere

Nevertheless, she decided to challenge the adversity, and so accepted the invitation.

"There's this thing that you have to be some supermodel walking out in your lingerie right after giving birth, which is ridiculous. Millions and millions of women have had babies for thousands of years. It's the most natural thing in the world. You get bigger for a period of time and then you lose the weight."—Tia Carrere

Losing the weight, however, also caused a little trouble for Tia.

"I lost it in front of twenty million people, every single week. I think that's what made it shocking. Then I had everybody saying, 'OK, what are you eating? How many hours a day are you dancing? I want to do that.'"—Tia Carrere

All she was really doing was following the intense *Dancing with the Stars* training schedule, which, in the end, proved to be incredibly positive.

"It was very gratifying getting back into shape so quickly."—Tia Carrere

Heather Mills, the Maverick

In season four viewers were treated to a *Dancing with the Stars* first—a contestant with a physical disability.

English animal rights campaigner Heather Mills accepted the invitation to compete on the show, despite having an artificial leg.

"Heather has twice the work that all the other celebrities have. Not only does she have to learn the steps, be on time, try to look graceful, but she has to balance on only one leg."
—Jonathan Roberts, Heather's dance partner.

Heather won praise for her courage but won fans for her superb dancing and infectious enthusiasm.

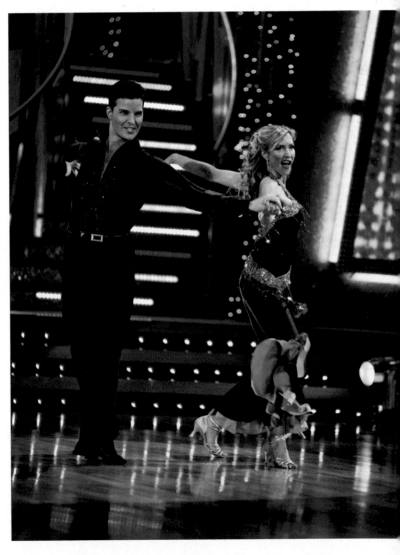

Using her disadvantage as an advantage, Heather made it her mission to inspire other amputees and anyone trying to overcome a disability, proving that they could get out there and dance, too.

"You have more guts than Rambo!"
—Bruno Tonioli, judge

During her run on the show, Heather refused to compromise her moves, and even wowed the judges with a tricky back walkover in her Mambo in show two.

Above all, not only was Heather an inspiration to viewers, she was also an inspiration to herself.

"A year ago, there's no way I would have ever believed that I would be dancing now."—Heather Mills

The Entertainers

Dancing with the Stars is not just about great dancing, but also about great performance and entertainment. There have been many characters on the show known more for their ability to make the audience laugh than their ability to twirl, and none more so than George Hamilton and Jerry Springer.

George Hamilton, the Comedian

By no means the master of technique, George chose to excite the judges with his power of entertainment in the Paso Doble.

"I'll go out laughing, but I'll certainly go out trying."
—George Hamilton

Basing his character on a part he had played in the spoof *Zorro, the Gay Blade,* he donned a mask and cape and pleased the judges with his amusing performance.

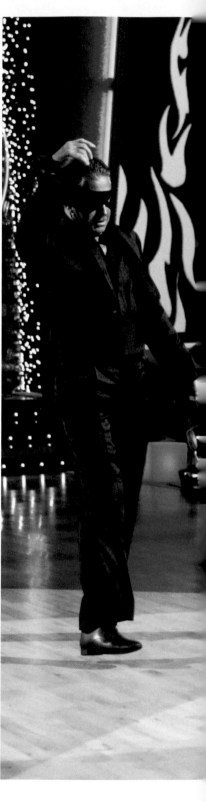

Judges' Comments

Len Goodman: *"What it lacked in technique, it made up for in entertainment."*

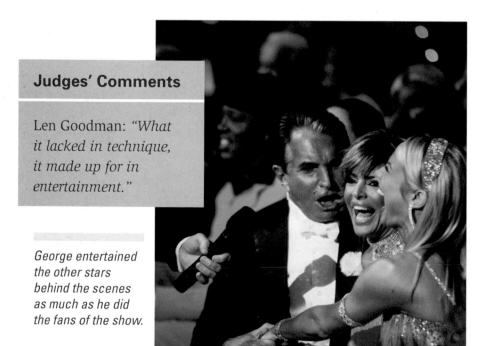

George entertained the other stars behind the scenes as much as he did the fans of the show.

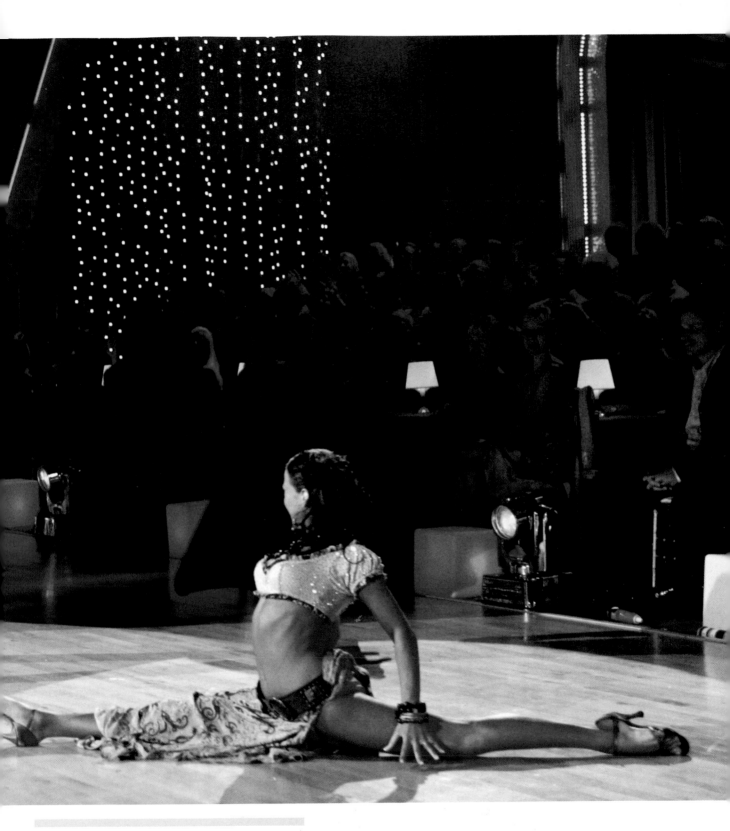

Zorro approaches his victim in a Paso Doble with
fantastic character created by George and Edyta.

Jerry Springer, the Character Actor

The secret to Jerry's performances was the amount of character he infused the dances with. Much of the credit must go to the humorous choreography put together by his partner, Kym Johnson, but Jerry took pains to really establish a character and a story.

"When I was doing the Samba, I wanted to perform with my face and hands. I said to her, 'We have to keep attention away from my feet. We don't have a prayer if they're looking at my feet. So I'll try to put on a show from the shoulders up.' I wanted to be over-the-top. I was thinking Lucille Ball, Red Skelton, Jerry Lewis—slapstick to the beat of the dance, so I would still respect the dance itself. That probably turned out to be our best performance." —Jerry Springer

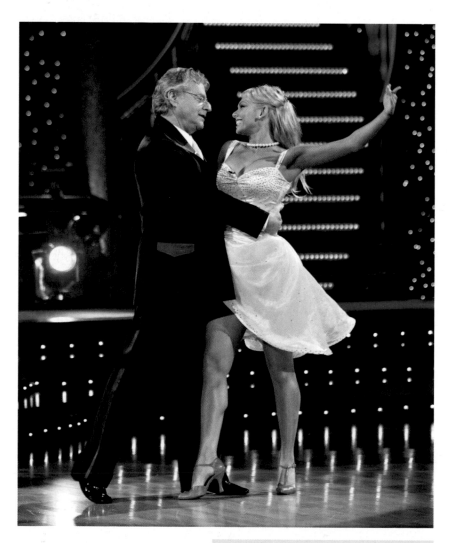

Jerry showing his daughter Katie that he was ready to Waltz on her wedding day.

The cheeky carnival Samba, and this Paso in which Jerry played the first matador to be afraid of the bull, were highlights of the season.

In addition, much of Jerry's motivation to take part in the show was to learn to dance the Waltz for his daughter Katie's wedding. It was especially moving because he also danced it to "Tennessee Waltz," a song he used to listen to as a child with his parents.

"This was going to be the biggest single moment in Katie's life. Therefore it became the most important moment in my life. I wanted it to be perfect. And the fact is, it was." —Jerry Springer

At the end of the performance, he hugged his daughter, reducing Carrie Ann to tears.

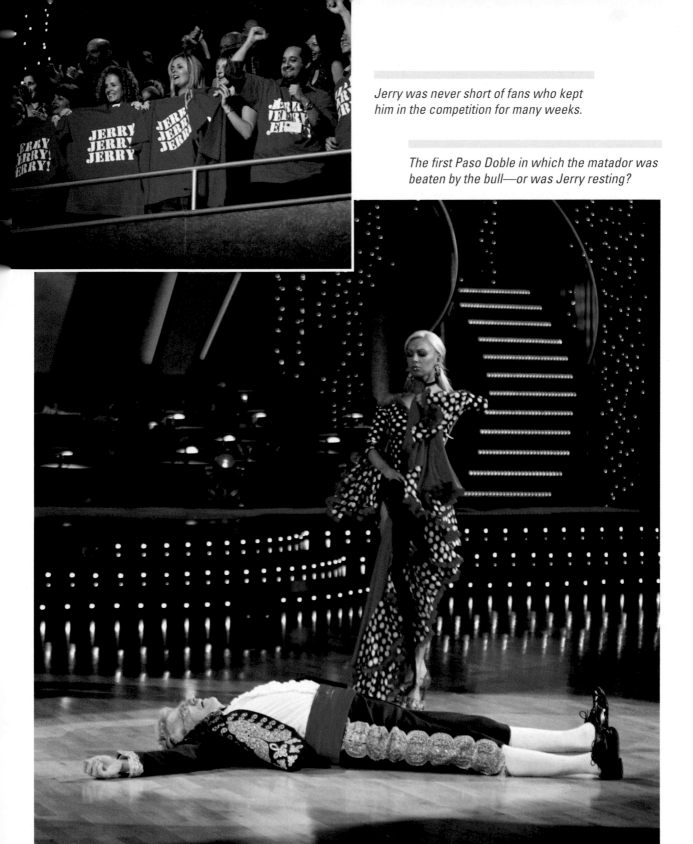

Jerry was never short of fans who kept him in the competition for many weeks.

The first Paso Doble in which the matador was beaten by the bull—or was Jerry resting?

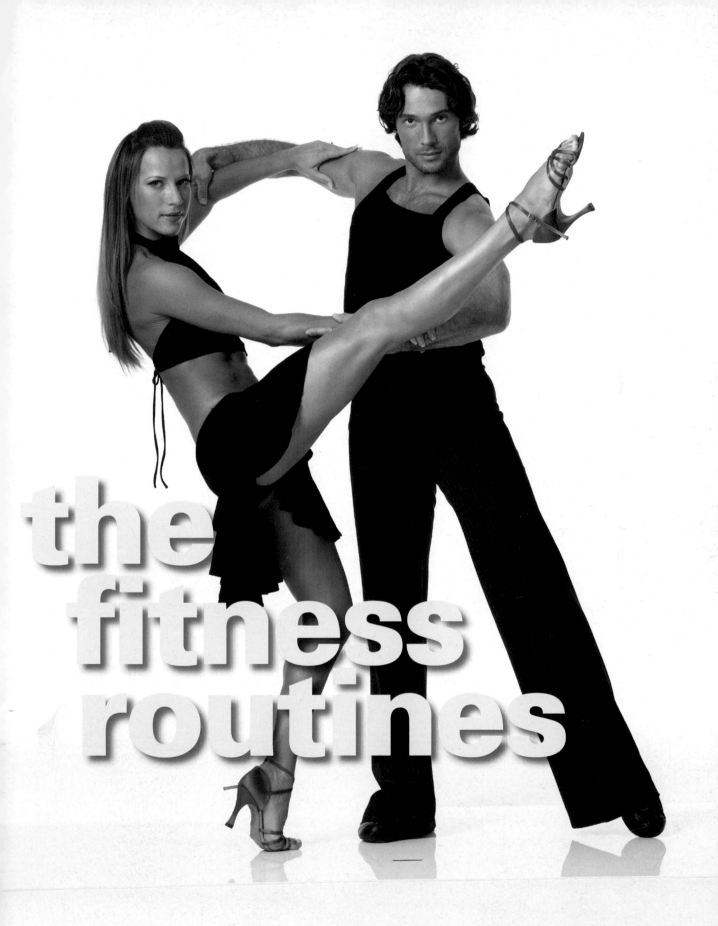

the
fitness
routines

introduction

THERE'S NO DENYING IT. Not only are the show's professional instructors great dance artists, but they also have amazing physiques. And if there is any doubt about the potential and effectiveness of ballroom dancing as a body-shaping form of exercise, look at those celebrity contestants whose overall physical appearance and strength have gone from "OK" and "so-so" to "Wow, wow!" In fact, sometimes you can almost see the pounds and inches start coming off at the very beginning of a Samba routine.

How do dancers get that sculpted waistline, the capped shoulders, the curvaceous hips, the sexy-looking thighs—the great buns?

If you are hoping for a secret formula, there isn't one. Well, not exactly.

The performers on *Dancing with the Stars* spend many hours and weeks rehearsing and practicing. That alone burns a lot of calories. But long periods of sheer calorie-burning physical activity are not strictly what sculpts the dancers' bodies. There are several other contributing factors.

Among them are strength training, flexibility training, core awareness and control, rhythmic pacing, correct posture and body alignment, and coordination. It is no surprise that all these factors are integral foundation elements of most forms and styles of dance—classical ballet, modern dance, jazz dance, folkloric dance, ballroom dance, etc.

Needless to say, most forms and styles of dance have different levels of performance. Ballroom dancing, for example, is performed not only on several social levels, but also on a semi-professional level, a professional level, an exhibition level, etc.

Ballroom dancing also features two different styles of performance: the American style and the international style. The latter is the style recognized at dance competitions worldwide. It is also the predominant style in the routines of the *Dancing with the Stars* contestants.

Generally, the higher the level of performance of an individual style of dance, the more the dancing will integrate movements and techniques characteristic of other styles. Consequently, today's ballroom-dance pros have to be masters of many different dance skills. They lift. They drop. They kick. They spin and swirl in fractions of a beat of music. Their hips no longer move exclusively in opposition to their traveling leg; they rotate, undulate, bump, and grind in all directions.

Their spines no longer mirror *Swan Lake* elegance, though they still can; they are strong as steel and flexible as a rubber band. Their feet need to be as strong and flexible as a springboard. Yet, they need to move softly and gracefully as well. To accomplish all that, the ballroom dancers on *Dancing with the Stars* not only train and work hard; they also train and work smart by integrating various styles of exercise into their workout routines.

Exercise? Isn't ballroom dance enough of an exercise? Ballroom dance, even at a beginner's social level, is wonderful exercise as it incorporates two of the three types of exercise medically recommended for improving health and fitness levels. One is strength training, which ballroom dancing provides through its dynamic use of major muscle groups. The other is flexibility, which involves the improvement and maintenance of joint range of motion.

The third major exercise component is cardiovascular exercise. Ballroom dancing per se, especially at a social level, does not qualify as cardiovascular exercise, one of the key elements of exercise in weight control.

The chapters in this section of the book feature a select group of exercises modeled by two pros from *Dancing with the Stars*, Alec Mazo and Edyta Sliwinska. Some of the exercises are simple and short. But most of the exercises comprise a sequence of individual movements, performed one after the other, structured to target the muscles or muscle groups most responsible for the execution of those movements.

In other words, just as in dance, you are getting various parts of your body to work together as one. And also as in dance, the focus of each sequence is the correct execution of each individual movement and a seamless flow between individual movements. Quality over quantity!

introduction

In addition, note that each exercise sequence is more intense than the previous one. Hence, it's recommended that you do them in progressive order.

Regardless, we offer many workout choices: You can integrate into your regular workout schedule an entire sequence of exercises that target an area of the body you feel needs the most attention; you can choose just one exercise from each sequence; or you can choose to do all the sequences as one continuous workout.

The sequences are grouped into four categories, plus warm-ups and stretches. Each of them is loosely related to the dances in the *Dancing with the Stars Cardio Dance DVD*. They are The Dancer's Warm-up; Paso Doble Arms and Shoulders; The Dancer's Abs and Core; Paso Doble Thighs, Buns, and Hips; Jive Dancing: Quick Feet and Great Legs; and Cool-down Stretches.

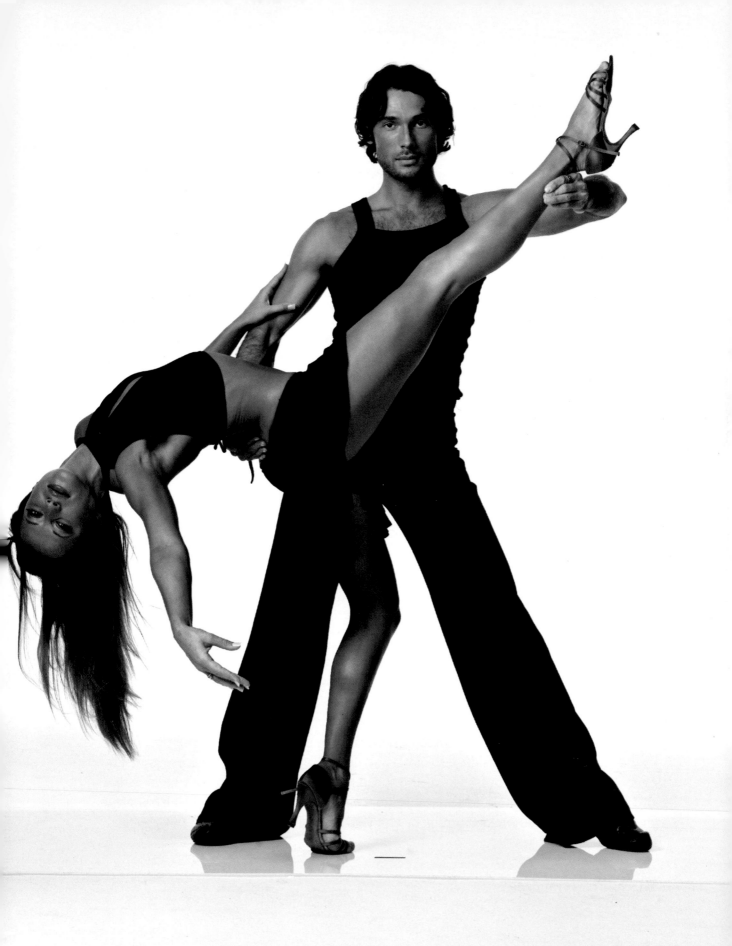

the dancer's warm-up

THE MAIN OBJECTIVE of warming-up is to increase the muscles' oxygen intake and to elevate the heart rate a couple of notches up to training speed. There are various ways in which to warm up.

Some are categorized as passive. For example, stretching the hamstring muscles by placing one foot on a surface that is at least calf height, then bending the torso over toward the leg, is referred to as a passive static stretch.

Other warm-ups are categorized as dynamic. For example, the combination of reaching out with the arms, circling them, and bending the knees into a squat is a series of dynamic movements in which various muscle groups contract to produce the action, while other muscle groups (antagonists) expand in order to stabilize the action.

Most dancers warm up before and cool down after a performance. Most performing-art dances—ballet, jazz, modern—start with a warm-up period. Any warm-up period should consist of movements or exercises that are specific to the type of physical activity the body is about to be subjected to.

For example, if you are going for a jog, starting with a fast-paced walk that progresses into a slow run and then into a jogging pace is the ideal way to get started, especially if you haven't jogged in a couple of days. If you are weight training and are about to start a bench press, doing a few reps with a light weight is a good idea before you start packing on the weight plates.

Because dance involves moving many muscle groups and joints in a variety of ways, a dance warm-up generally consists of various movements that strengthen muscles and increase range of motion (flexibility).

The Dancer's Warm-up that follows consists of individual movements and movement sequences designed to blend and flow in and out of one another. Start slow until you memorize each of the movements and are able to link them into a routine that should last no more than seven or eight minutes. It's also a great routine to start your morning or end your day with.

exercise 1: salutation stretch

This exercise is fashioned after a sequence created by one of the most famous dance teachers of Broadway musical stars of all time, "Luigi," and is performed by dancers all over the world. It's a sequence of four different movements that combine rib cage, hip, and spine isolations that get opposing sides of the body moving and stretching at the same time. There's no area of the body that's left untouched by this combination.

first movement

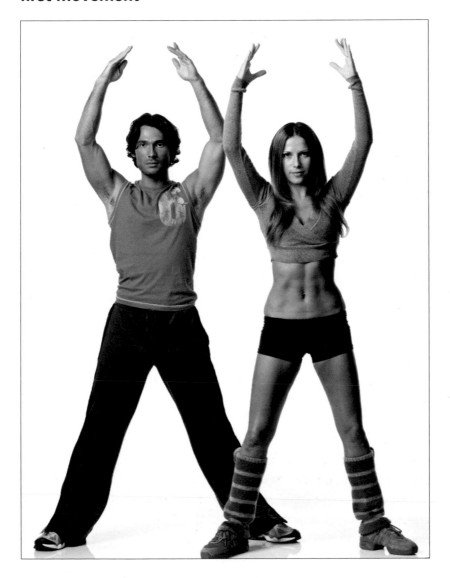

Starting position: Stand with your feet wide apart and with your arms reaching upward above your head. Keep your core muscles firmly held and your shoulders down.

the dancer's warm-up

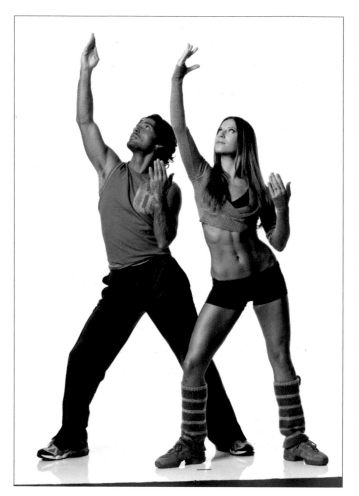

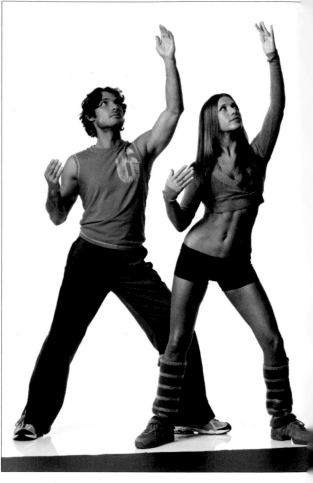

Bow and Arrow stretch:

1. *Reach up with your right hand as high as you can, allowing your right shoulder and the right side of your rib cage to stretch upward. Bend your left arm at the elbow.*

2. At the same time, let your right knee bend over the right toes and your left hip move sideways to the left. This movement feels like pointing a bow upward and holding it with one hand high above the head, while the other hand is pulling down on the arrow.

Alternate right and left sides four times.

second movement

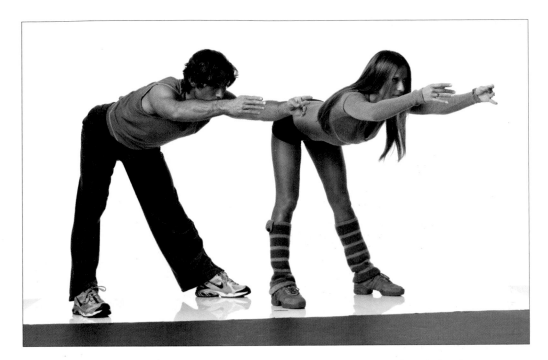

Forward Bend: *Bend forward at the waist, keeping your knees slightly bent—never locked. Keep your abdominal muscles firm. The feel of this movement should be one of elongation. As your torso reaches a horizontal position parallel to the floor, you should feel as if your hands, neck, and shoulders are reaching forward while your tailbone is reaching out back.*

third movement

The Rag Doll: *Let your knees continue to bend in the direction of the toes as you continue bending down from the waist toward the floor. Let your arms hang freely from each shoulder, and bring your chin in toward your chest.*

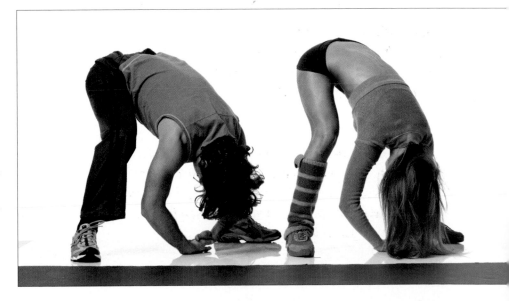

the dancer's warm-up

fourth movement

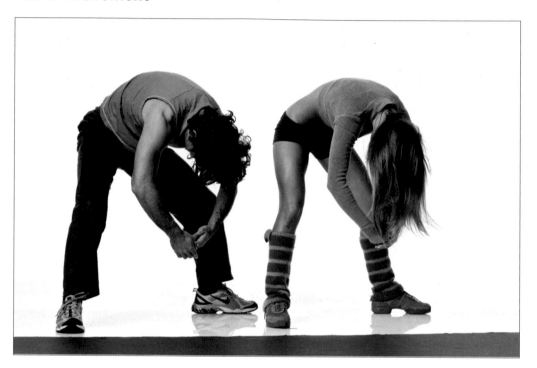

Rising Tower:

1. As you straighten your legs, start rolling upward from your lower spine. Take your time and focus on each vertebra, visualizing each one being placed on top of the others until you are standing straight.

2. Then continue the movement by taking the arms back to the same position you started the entire combination with.

Repeat the entire combination two to four times.

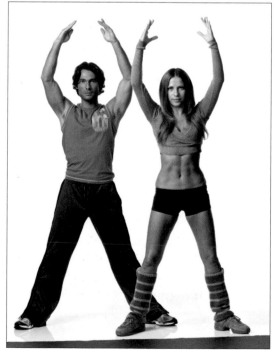

exercise 2: upper body stretch

This is both a warm-up and a great releaser of stress for the shoulders, upper back, and chest.

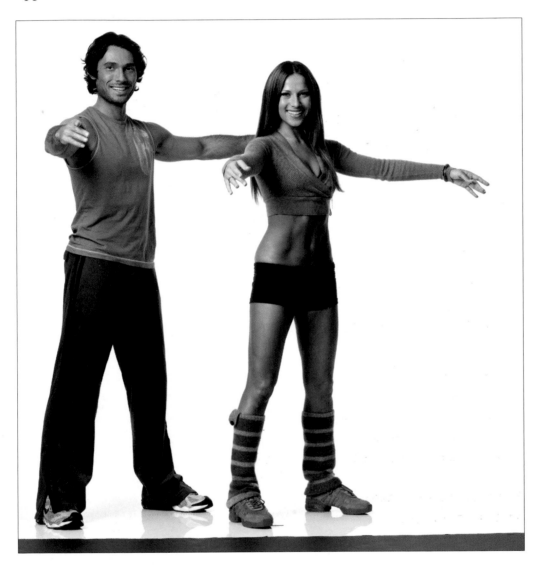

Starting position: Stand with your legs apart and arms to the sides. Feel as if your arms are reaching out to the left and right corners of the wall you are facing instead of to the walls that are to the left and to the right of you. Your shoulder blades should feel as far apart from each other as possible rather than pinned toward each other. Take a deep breath.

the dancer's warm-up

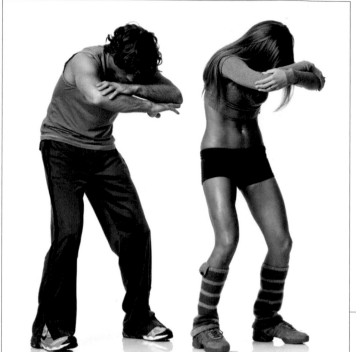

first movement

Bend your knees slightly. Pull your belly button in toward your spine. Bring your arms to the front, rounding your back and bringing your chin in toward your chest. Exhale.

second movement

Return to your standing position, bringing both arms around to the sides and out behind you with the palms of both hands facing each other. Pin your shoulder blades together, allowing your chest to stretch and expand. Keep your core muscles firm to avoid arching your lower back.

Exhale.

Repeat contraction and extension two to four times.

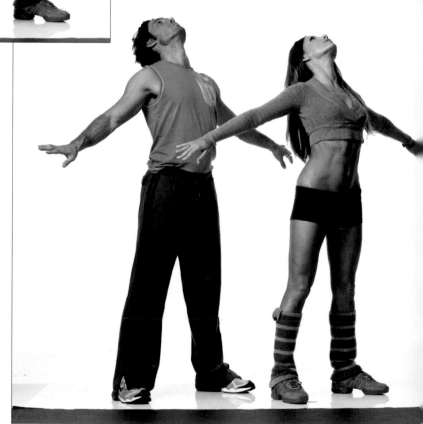

exercise 3: two-way lateral stretch

Starting position: Stand with your feet together and your weight on the right foot.

first movement

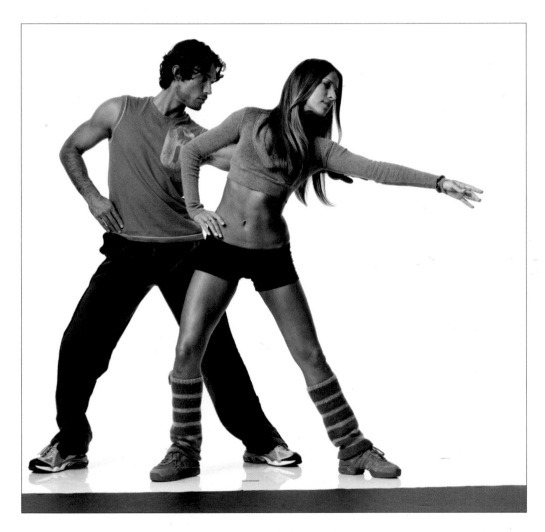

1. As you bend your right knee, bend to the left from the waist, extending both the left arm and the left leg out to the side.

2. Slide your right hand up the opposite side of the upper body. The feeling here is not one of bending to the left but of elongating the right side of the upper body.

the dancer's warm-up

second movement

Use your right thigh to push off the floor in order to bring the body back to a standing position. As you push off, keep raising your left arm sideways and upward, elongating the left side of the body and leaning to the right from the waist.

From this position, repeat the movement two to four times before changing weight and doing the same on the other side.

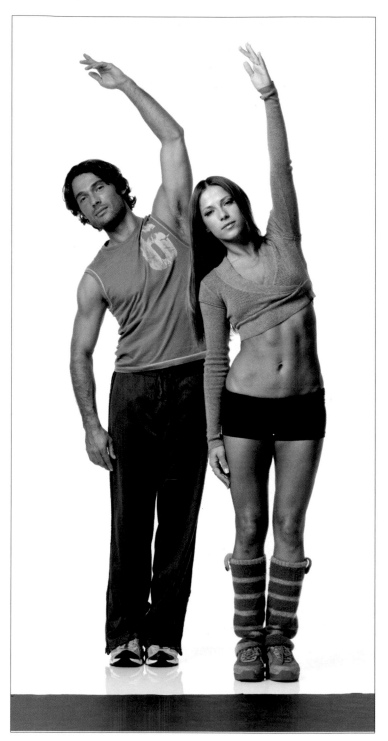

exercise 4: three-point isolations

In dance we move the body as a complete unit as often as we move its individual or isolated parts. Latin dances like the Samba, the Cha-cha, and the Mambo and rhythm dances like the Jive feature lots of isolated movements. As simple as isolations may look, they actually require a lot of concentration. They also call for core control. The abdominal muscles must be kept firmly engaged in order to keep the body's weight evenly distributed between both feet while isolating movements are being performed.

first movement: shoulder isolations

Visually, this movement shows the shoulders moving up and forward. However, the mechanics of this movement start with the shoulder blade.

Starting position: Feet slightly apart with knees bent. Place hands on the waist with elbows pointing outward.

1. Make a forward circular motion with your left shoulder by raising your left shoulder blade, then extending it forward, a protracting movement.

2. Then, reverse this movement by drawing in the shoulder blade and protracting it back in place. Repeat the same movements with the other shoulder.

Alternate between shoulders for four to six repetitions.

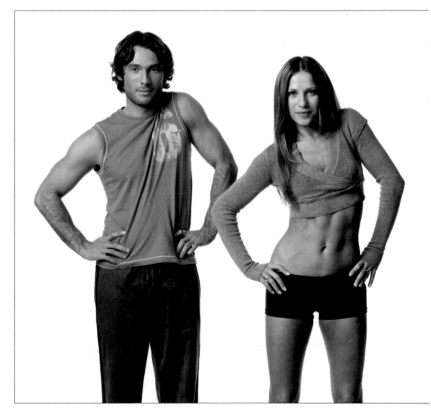

the dancer's warm-up

second movement: rib cage isolations

Latin dances are known for their hip action. In dance, this action is called "Cuban motion." It involves the rhythmic synchronization of the knees, hips, and rib cage during a weight-shifting action. In this particular exercise, the objective is to move the entire rib cage to the left or the right without allowing the body's weight to shift from one leg to the other.

Starting position: Feet shoulder-width apart and parallel. Hands on waist.

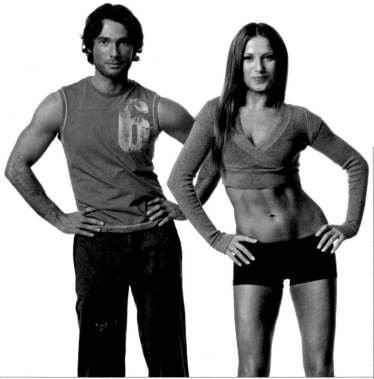

◀ *1. Move the rib cage as far to the right as you can, then back to the center.*

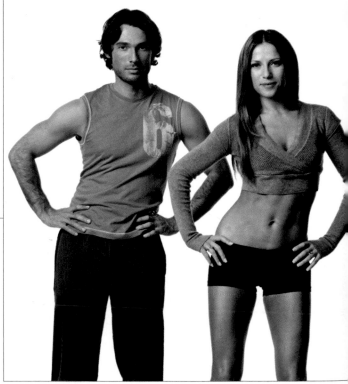

▶ *2. Move the rib cage as far to the left as you can, then back to the center.*

Continue shifting from right to left for ten to twelve repetitions.

third movement: hip isolations

Starting position: Feet should remain shoulder-width apart with knees slightly bent and pointing toward the toes. The body's weight should be equally distributed between both feet.

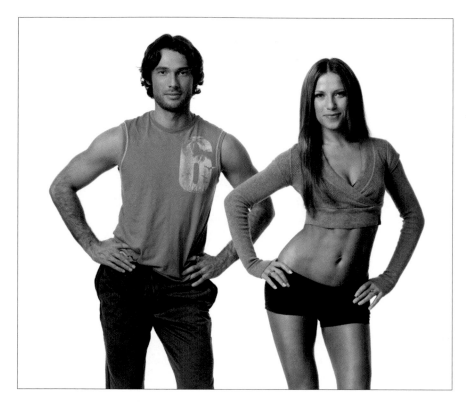

1. Shift your right hip over to the right side. As you do so, your right knee will start to straighten, although never fully. Keep your lower abdominal muscles firm and engaged.

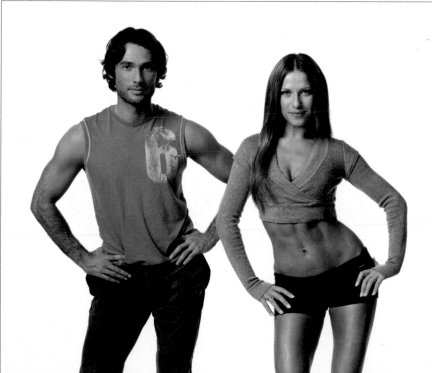

2. Repeat the movement with your left hip.

Continue shifting from right to left for ten to twelve repetitions.

the dancer's warm-up

exercise 5: isolation challenge

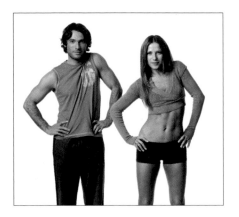

After repeating all three isolations a few times, see if you can combine them all into one sequence, i.e., right and left shoulder isolation, followed by right and left rib-cage isolation, and then right and left hip isolation.

Repeat eight to ten times.

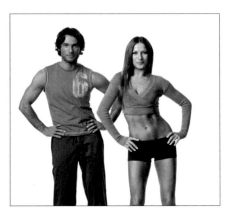

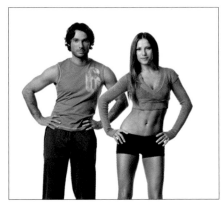

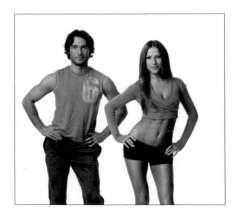

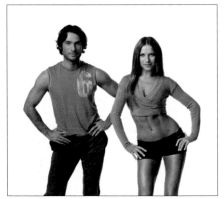

exercise 6: round the globe

This exercise sequence consists of two simultaneous movement sequences that combine a dynamic stretch of the entire upper torso with a curtsy-like movement, frequently referred to as a "skater's squat," that works the muscles of the buttocks, hips, and thighs. Once the full sequence is completed on one side of the body, it is then reversed to the opposite side of the body.

Starting Position: Stand with feet shoulder-width apart, with knees flexed and arms extended downward alongside the body.

first movement: reach and extend

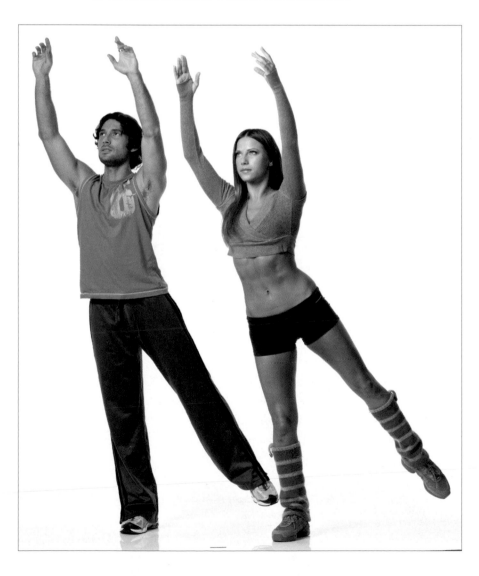

1. Shift your weight over to the right foot and turn your upper body toward the right corner of the room.

2. From their extended position, swing the arms out to the right and up toward the upper right corner of the room, reaching for the point where ceiling and walls meet.

3. As you reach, extend the left leg diagonally behind you. Point the left foot. You should feel as if your hands and your left foot are each at two opposite ends of an elastic band that's being stretched out and tautly held.

the dancer's warm-up

second movement: bend and squat (curtsy)

It takes three simultaneously executed motions to complete the Second Movement of this exercise.

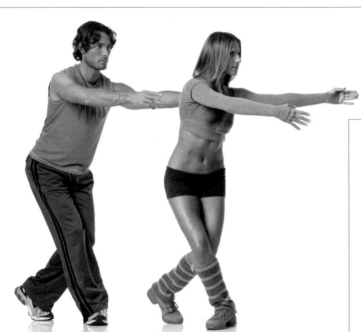

◀ *1. From the outstretched position, start swinging both arms over to the left upper corner of the room. Keep you weight balanced over the right leg and keep the left leg extended diagonally behind you.*

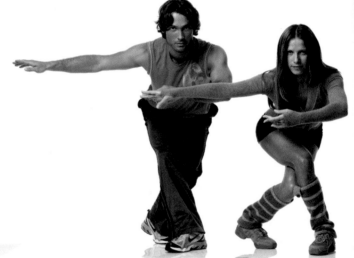

▶ *2. As your arms continue to swing left and downward, reaching the level of your shoulders, bend the left knee and place it right behind the right knee. The front of your left thigh should be directly behind the back of your right thigh.*

3. As you continue to swing the arms from left to right, (1) bend forward at the waist, keeping your upper torso long; (2) bend your knees, pressing one thigh against the other and move your buttocks back towards the floor. During this movement, you should feel that the buttocks and the upper back are both moving in opposite directions. This is a wonderful warm-up stretch for the major and minor muscles along the spine.

From this position, come up and step to the left with your left foot and start the entire sequence on that foot.

exercise 7: standing curl and layout

Starting position: Stand with feet shoulder-width apart and arms fully extended alongside the body.

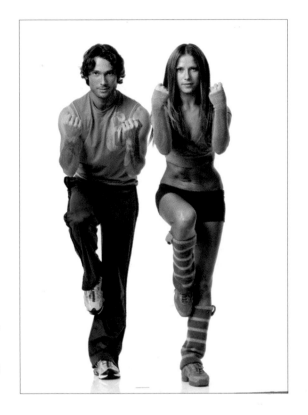

first movement: standing curl

Lean forward from the waist as you bend your elbows and bring your right knee toward your chest. Tighten the core muscles as you curl in.

second movement: layout

1. From the curling position, take a large step to the right. Extend your left leg out to the side and let your arms stretch out toward the sides of the room.

2. From this layout position, come straight up on your right leg and perform the Standing Curl with your left knee, followed by a layout to the left side.

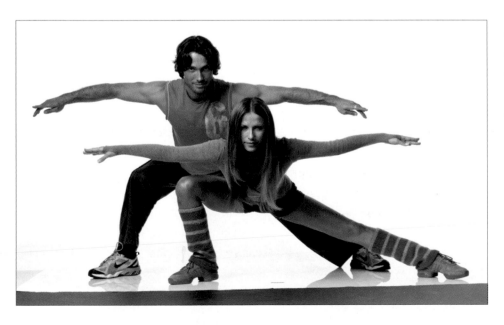

Alternate between left and right for a total of eight reps—four on each side.

paso doble arms and shoulders

IN ADDITION to being a partnered dance, the Paso Doble is also the name of a Spanish style of musical composition that dates back to the eighteenth century and was played at military ceremonies: Marching soldiers stepped on the strongest beat of the music, the downbeats. Then, instead of taking another step on the next beat, the upbeat, they tapped their moving foot, next to their supporting foot, letting the beat go by and waiting for the next downbeat to take another step. This step followed by a toe tap became known as a Paso Doble, or "double step."

The Paso Doble is also known as "el Baile de los Toreadores" or "the Dance of the Bullfighters." When the Paso Doble became associated with bullfights is not exactly known. But it is widely accepted that it was around the nineteenth century that small bands started to play Paso Dobles during the bullfighters' ceremonial entrance into the arena. Over the years, many Paso Dobles have been composed as tributes to legendary bullfighters—and even to bulls who put up such a good fight their lives were ultimately spared.

It was not until the late 1920s that the Paso Doble started to also become known as a social dance, which eventually evolved into one of the international-style competitive rhythm dances. One thing is certain. There is a huge difference between the social-level Paso Doble and its brother, the competition-level Paso Doble.

Socially, this is a very easy dance to learn and to do. Most of its signature patterns consist of sequences of marchlike steps danced in groups of eight to sixteen beats of music. For the most part, the female's dance patterns are the mirror opposite of the male's.

On the other hand, the competition- and exhibition-level Paso Doble—or "Paso," as many professionals refer to it—is a highly spirited and intricate dance. For years, many people have described this dance as one in which the male plays the role of the bullfighter and the female that of his cape. Dancers combine standardized ballroom-dance patterns with patterns and movements from other dance styles, especially Flamenco.

In this photograph, Edyta's movement and Alec's pose symbolize a matador challenging the bull with his cape.

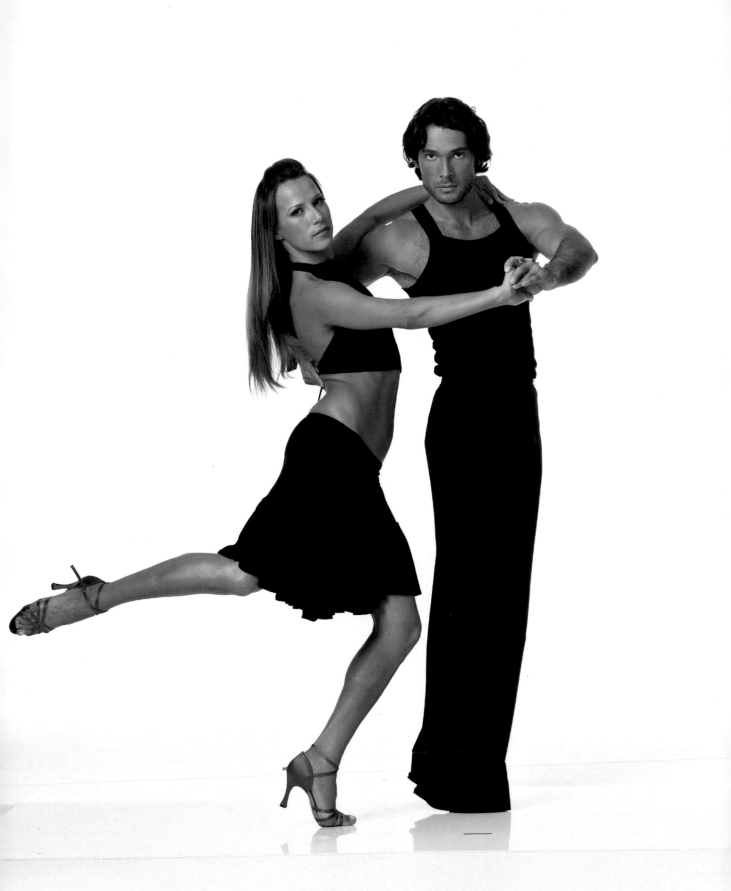

paso doble arms and shoulders

Lunges, knee crawls, backbends, high kicks, and complex foot movements stylized with Flamenco stomps and kicks are but a few of the moves that characterize and embellish competition-level choreography. Needless to say, these moves call for extensive training and practice. They also call for strong knees and thighs, a firm abdominal core, flexibility in the hips and spine, and shoulder and biceps muscles that are as strong as they look sexy and graceful. And especially on the dance floor, the moves call for a bit of matador-like attitude.

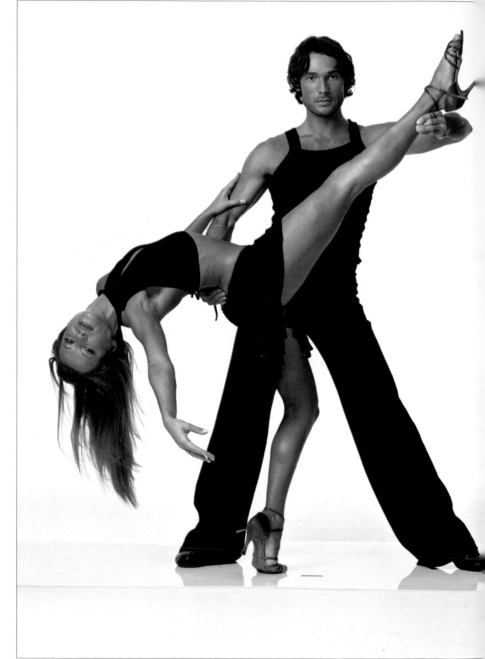

paso doble arms

The Paso Doble is a forceful-looking dance. No matter how much macho showmanship is displayed during a dance, weak-looking arms will detract from it. Yet a male dancer's arms should be and look strong without looking like the arms of a power lifter. Alec's arms are perfectly sculpted and in proportion with his powerful dancer's body.

The following biceps and triceps exercises use the pull of gravity to add more resistance to the weights. The focus of each exercise should not be the bending action of the arm—the contraction of the focused muscle group—but the body posture and alignment that are maintained throughout the exercise. Done with the correct body alignment, these exercises will also engage the abdominal core.

Women should start these exercises with the three-pound dumbbells (d-bells). Men should start with five-pound d-bells. The maximum weight that should be used is twelve pounds.

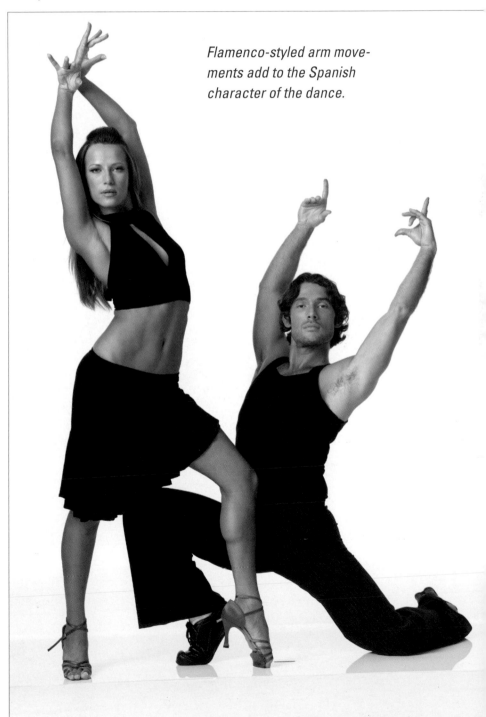

Flamenco-styled arm movements add to the Spanish character of the dance.

paso doble arms and shoulders

exercise 1: biceps curl combination

This exercise alternates between a hammer curl and an across-the-body curl.

Starting position: Stand tall with feet shoulder-width apart. Keep knees at a slightly bent angle, with shoulders down and core muscles firmly held. Start with the arms extended alongside the body, d-bells held in a tight grip.

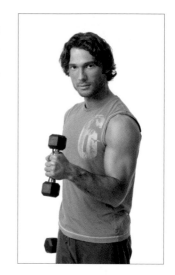

▶ *1. Bend the elbow keeping it fixed (stabilized) against its side of the body. Continue bending it while lifting the d-bell toward the right shoulder and feeling the biceps muscle contract. Slowly lower it back to its starting position.*

◀ *2. Repeat the same movement with the right arm. Keep the core muscles engaged!*

◀ *3. Lift the left d-bell across the front of the body. Focus on contracting the left biceps muscle.*

Return to the starting position.

▶ *Repeat the same movement with the right arm.*

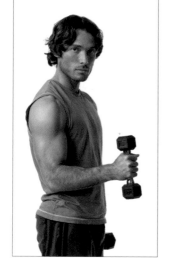

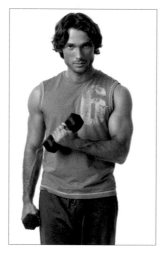

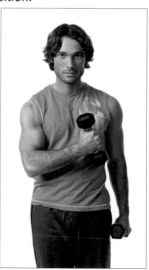

A set consists of one hammer curl for each arm and one across-the-body curl for each arm.

Women should start with six to eight sets. Men should start with ten to twelve sets. If the last two sets are easy to do, increase the weight of the d-bells.

exercise 2: pilates curls

This biceps curl has been credited to the late Joseph Pilates, whose pioneering work in rehabilitating the bodies of injured ballet dancers at his New York City studio has become one of today's most popular exercise systems. A main focus of any Pilates exercise is body alignment through the constant engagement of the abdominal core.

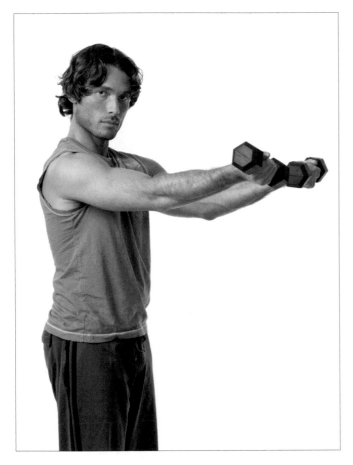

Starting position: Stand with feet shoulder-width apart. Shoulders are down and core muscles firmly engaged.

◀ *1. Extend both dumbbell-holding arms in front of the body with palms of the hands facing up.*

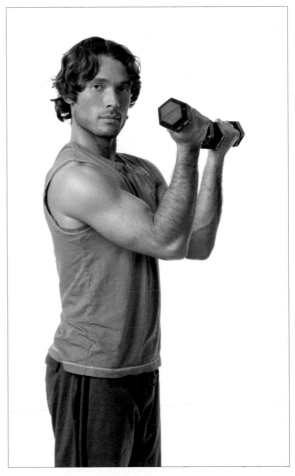

▶ *2. Keeping the upper arms as horizontal (parallel to the floor) as possible, curl the d-bells toward you. Doing this calls for further engagement of the abdominal core. Do not let the shoulders rise through the curling motion. Take the arms back to their fully extended position.*

Eight to ten reps.

paso doble arms and shoulders

exercise 3: strong-man curls

Here again the core muscles are used to stabilize the upper body.

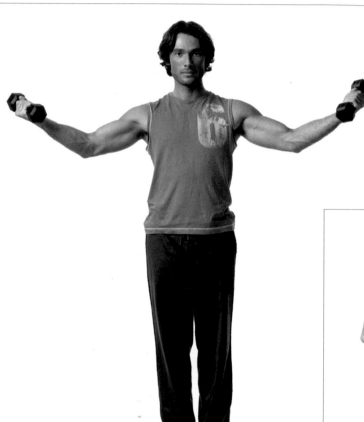

◀ *1. Starting position: Extend the arms out to the sides without locking the elbows. Keep the shoulders down and the shoulder blades as far apart as possible, hence keeping your upper back in its natural rounded position.*

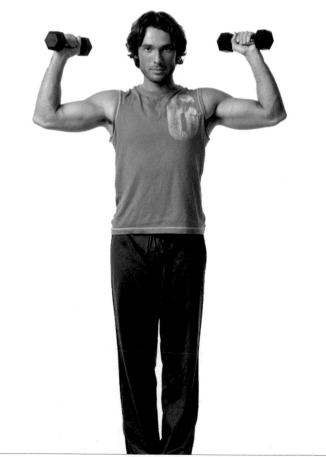

▶ *2. Keeping both upper arms horizontal and parallel to the floor, bend the elbows as you bring the d-bells toward you. Return to the starting position.*

Ten to twelve reps.

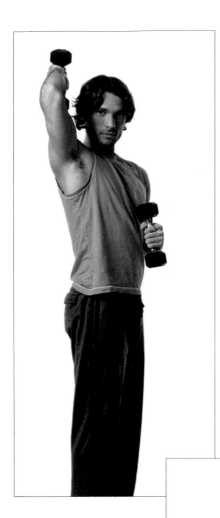

exercise 4: triceps press

This wonderful triceps sculptor also engages the shoulder muscles.

Starting position: Hold the d-bell behind the neck. Make sure not to place the bent elbow too far back. It should be pointing to the two o'clock position and never to the three o'clock.

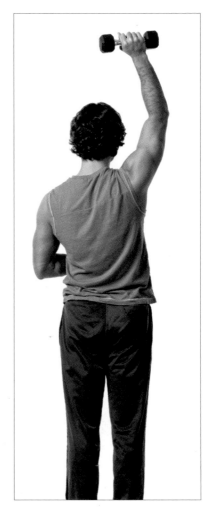

▶ *1. Extend the arm upward, but never as far as letting the elbow lock.*

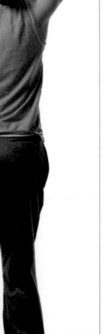

◀ *2. Lower the d-bell back behind the neck. Keep the functioning elbow stabilized in a fixed position through the extending and bending motion.*

Ten to twelve reps on each side.

paso doble arms and shoulders

exercise 5: triceps dip

This exercise requires the use of a work-out bench or a stable chair. If you use a chair, place it against a wall or a surface that will not allow the chair to slide in any direction during the exercise. Do you recognize the chair in the picture?

Starting position: Place your hands on the front edge of the chair's seat, and place your feet far enough in front of the chair that you can bring your upper torso down in front of the seat. Notice how straight Alec keeps his back and his arms.

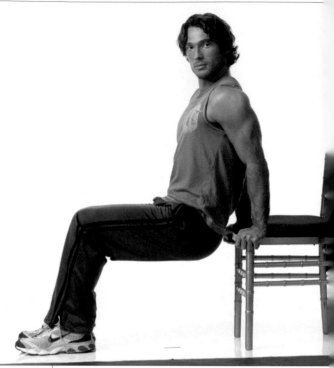

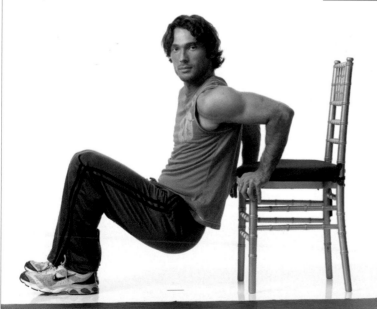

◀ *Lower your body by bending the elbows toward the back of the chair. You must focus on not letting the shoulders rise as you lower yourself or as you return back to your starting position.*

Ten to twelve dips.

exercise 6: plank push-ups

This is a very effective exercise executed from a plank position. In addition to engaging the core muscles, it also gets the shoulder and chest muscles into action.

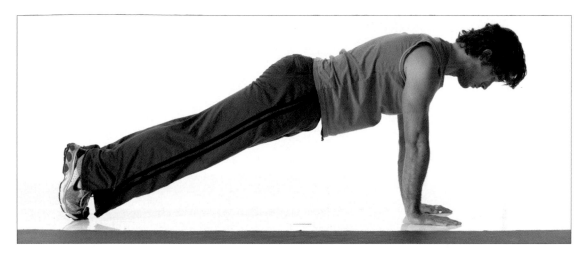

Starting position: Just as you see in this picture, position your body facedown toward the floor with arms fully extended. Hands should be directly under the shoulders with fingers facing forward.

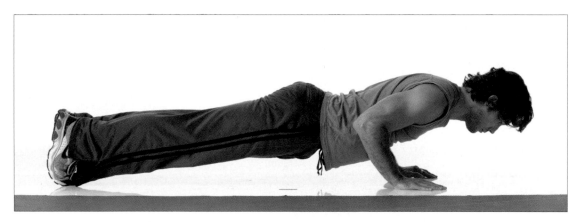

Lower your body toward the floor by bending the elbows. Hold the position for at least five counts. Keep the elbows close to the sides of the body. Aim for achieving a ninety-degree angle between the upper arm and forearm. Press your body back to starting position.

Eight to ten push-ups.

paso doble arms and shoulders

exercise 7: yoga stretch

Commonly known as a Downward Dog yoga stretch, this is a good movement to do after the Plank Push-up.

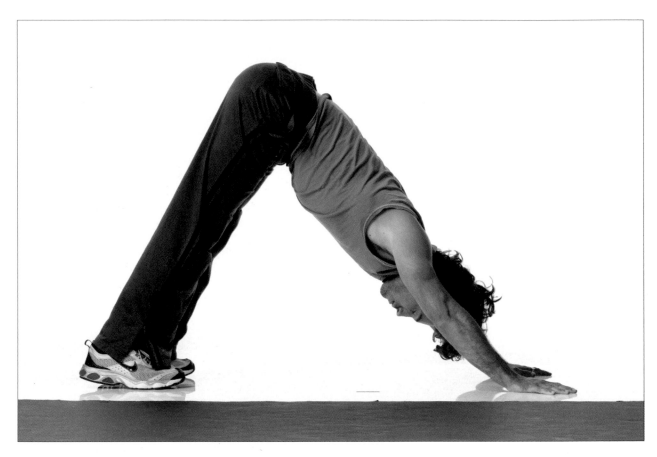

1. Starting from your last Plank Push-up, raise your hips up to the ceiling. Your aim is to form an inverted V with your body. Try bringing your heels as close to the ground as possible. Keep pulling up on the thigh muscles as you work to align your arms, shoulders, and spine all in one straight line.

2. Hold the position for a few seconds. Gradually and slowly come back up to a standing position.

paso doble shoulders

Many Paso Doble patterns call for dancers to maintain a steady dance frame. This is not easy to do, especially during patterns that weave in and out of dance positions at a fast pace. Having weak shoulder and upper-back muscles make keeping a correct frame even more difficult. In addition, the Paso Doble features many movements in which the arms strike various poses one after the other. These sudden changes of position require shoulder strength and good range of motion.

Edyta's shoulders are both strong and graceful. The following arm and shoulder exercises she's modeled for you have been selected for their simplicity and

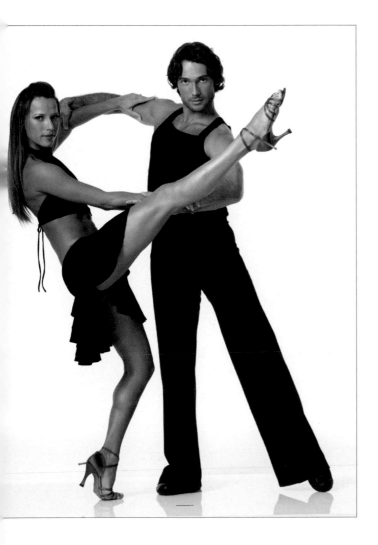

In this photograph, the arms of Alec and Edyta are forming a perfectly held open "dance frame." Simply put, a dance frame is the position held by the arms of a dance team during the course of their dance. Dance frames vary according to the dance being performed. But without strong shoulder and upper back muscles, maintaining any characteristic dance frame is difficult, especially during patterns that weave in and out of dance positions at a fast pace as it frequently happens in the Paso Doble. In addition, the Paso Doble features many movements during which the arms extend high above the head or behind the body. Sometimes, arms change from one extended position to another in just one beat of music. These sudden changes tax the shoulder and rotator cuff muscles.

paso doble arms and shoulders

proven results in increasing muscular strength and power without adding visible mass. The exercises should be done with three- to five-pound dumbbells to start with. As your arms and shoulders get stronger, and if you wish for a more sculpted look, you might want to increase the volume of the weights to eight to ten pounds, or you can increase the number of sets.

If you've never worked with weights before, one rule-of-thumb is to start with just ten to twelve reps of each exercise. Shoulders are delicate joints, so you should start with the lowest weight possible: three pounds. If during your first workout you can do twelve reps easily, you may consider increasing the weight.

It is always smart to keep a regular workout schedule of two or three times a week for at least three weeks before you start increasing the weight volume or the number of sets you do.

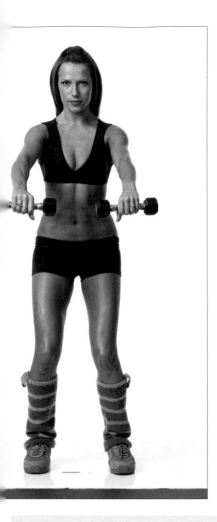

exercise 1: front raises

Nothing helps to shape the shoulders into sexy-looking caps and strengthen the muscles in the scapular area (i.e., the rotator-cuff group) like a combination of d-bell raises. If they are done slowly and with the correct body alignment, there's no need to use heavy weights. You can achieve a lot with three- and five-pound d-bells.

Starting position: Stand with feet shoulder-width apart. Knees should not be locked, and core muscles should be kept firm throughout. Shoulders are down. Dumbbells are held with the palms of the hands turned to face the floor.

◀ *1. Keeping the arms extended without locking the elbows, raise both arms to just above the belly button.*

2. Maintain that position for at least five seconds. Keep the dumbbells horizontal.

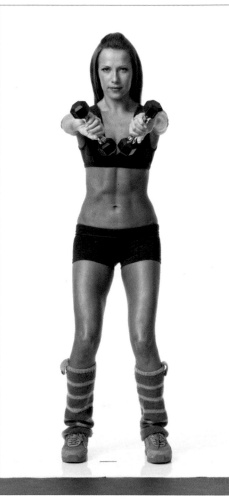

▶ *3. Then raise the arms to chest level, twisting the wrists inward toward each other. Visualize you are pouring two separate quarts of milk into a bowl.*

4. Bring the d-bells back down to the starting position.

Eight to twelve slow reps.

Correct Execution Tips

1. When doing raises—front or side—the shoulders should be kept down and relaxed. You can best achieve this by focusing on keeping your shoulder blades as far apart as possible, as well as keeping them down. If when doing this exercise you feel as though your shoulder blades want to rise, you might be lifting too much weight.

2. Keep your core muscles firm and slightly pulled in toward the spine. This will help prevent you from arching your lower back beyond its natural curve.

paso doble arms and shoulders

exercise 2: lateral raises

This exercise combines a turned-out leg squat and lateral d-bell raises.

Starting position: Stand with legs wide apart and slightly turned out from the hip. Hold the d-bells in front of the body and horizontal with palms facing the floor.

▶ *1. Raise the d-bells up to just above the level of the belly button. Hold that position for five seconds.*

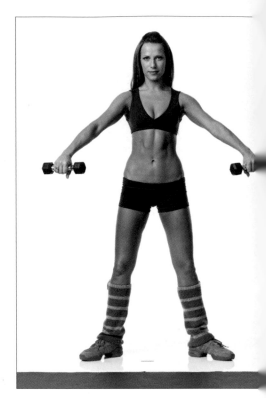

Correct Execution Tip

In dance, when arms are raised off to the side, it doesn't mean they are reaching out in the direction of a room's side walls. Taking the arms too far back, especially when holding weights, can harm the shoulder joints and the rotator-cuff muscles. You can achieve the correct body-to-arm alignment by thinking of the front of your body as squarely facing twelve o'clock. Then extend your right arm in the direction of two o'clock, and your left in the direction of ten o'clock.

▶ *2. Then raise the arms to chest level, twisting the wrists in toward each other (pouring milk) and bending the knees into a plié squat. Knees should move toward the toes of their corresponding feet.*

3. Return to the starting position slowly. In fact, this entire combination should be done slowly.

Eight to twelve slow reps.

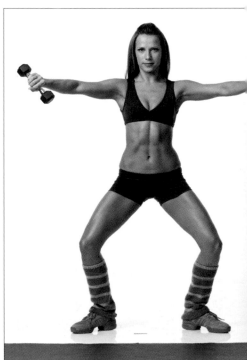

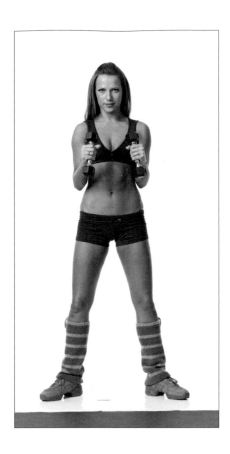

exercise 3: rotator toners

The rotator cuff is made up of four muscles that support and stabilize the shoulder joint. Circular arm motions, predominant in Latin dances, task the rotator cuff. Keeping these muscles strong is very important.

Starting position: Stand with feet shoulder-width apart. Keep your elbows bent and in a fixed position at each side of the body. Holding the d-bells vertical, keep the forearms horizontal and parallel to the floor.

▶ *1. Open the arms outward to about a forty-five-degree angle, rotating the forearm from its elbow-fixed point.*

2. Return to the starting position.

Ten to twelve reps.

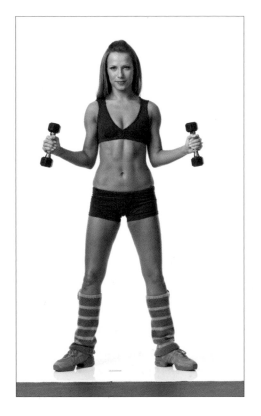

Optional position: This exercise is also very effective when performed with the body lying down sideways on the floor.

1. Holding the d-bell, place the elbow on the side of the rib cage farthest from the floor. Let the d-bell touch the floor.

2. Keep the elbow fixed in place at a ninety-degree angle.

3. Lift the d-bell straight up to a distance equal to one and a half times your body's width.

4. Bring the d-bell back to the floor.

Repeat this motion ten to twelve times. Rest for thirty seconds. Repeat again. Maximum weight load should be five pounds.

paso doble arms and shoulders

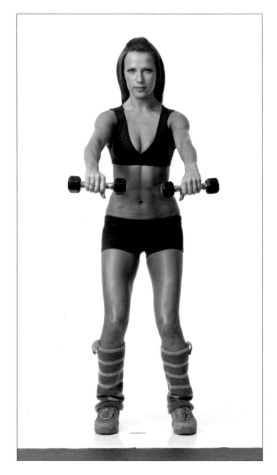

exercise 4: cape cappers

During one of the *Dancing with the Stars* competitions, Olympic gold medalist Apolo Anton Ohno danced a terrific Paso Doble in which he used his partner's skirt as if it were a bullfighter's cape, swirling it above his head and around his body. This type of dance movement taxes the muscles of the shoulders and upper back. The following exercise is designed to strengthen those areas and to help you get those sexy-looking shoulder caps. It consists of a 360-degree circular motion to the right and to the left performed with the arms extended, as if you were swirling a cape overhead.

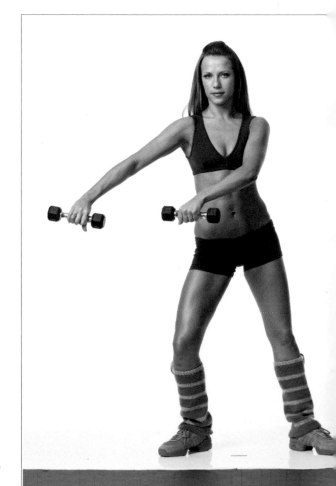

▲ Starting position: Stand with your feet apart and arms extended, holding d-bells with the palms of your hands facing the floor.

▶ *1. As you lunge to one side, swing your arms in the direction of your lunging foot.*

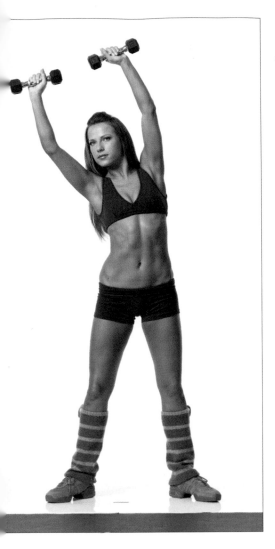

◀ 2. Continue the upward swing motion, straightening the legs as the arms reach their highest mark. The d-bells should be in your field of vision all the time, especially when your arms are at their highest point.

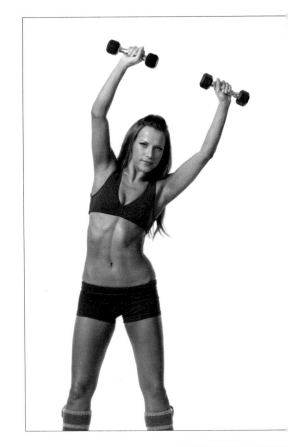

▶ 3. Let your upper body sway from the waist in the direction of the d-bells. Doing this engages the external oblique muscles of your core. Keep your shoulders from rising throughout this motion.

▶ 4. As you bring the d-bells down on the other side, completing the circle, lunge to the side.

Perform six to eight Cappers to the right and then to the left.

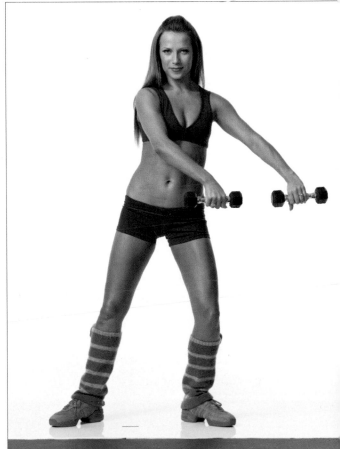

paso doble arms and shoulders

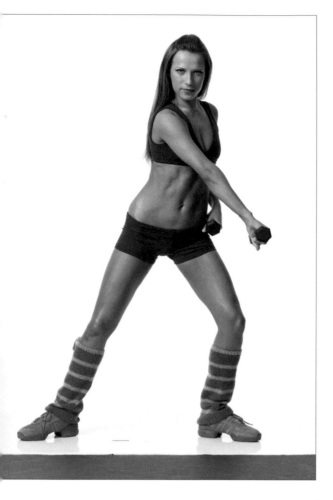

exercise 5: standing rows

This exercise is great for the front of the shoulders as well as for strengthening and sculpting the blades area.

Starting position: Stand with legs apart and with a slight turnout. Hold each d-bell alongside each hip.

◀ *1. Lunge to the left, extending your right arm across your body and over to the lunging foot. The palm of the right hand should be facing the floor. Keep your hips facing forward, but allow the entire right shoulder area to move toward the d-bell.*

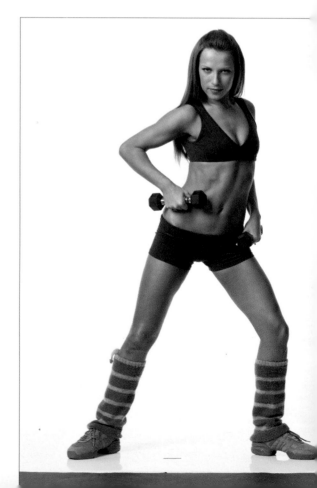

▶ *2. This next motion should resemble a sawing or rowing motion. Bring the d-bell back to its hip-level starting position. Focus on your right shoulder blade. It should be the motion of the shoulder blade retracting back into place that is bringing the right arm back to its starting position.*

Ten to twelve reps on each side.

exercise 6: shoulder stretch

After a good shoulder workout, this feels *sooo good.*

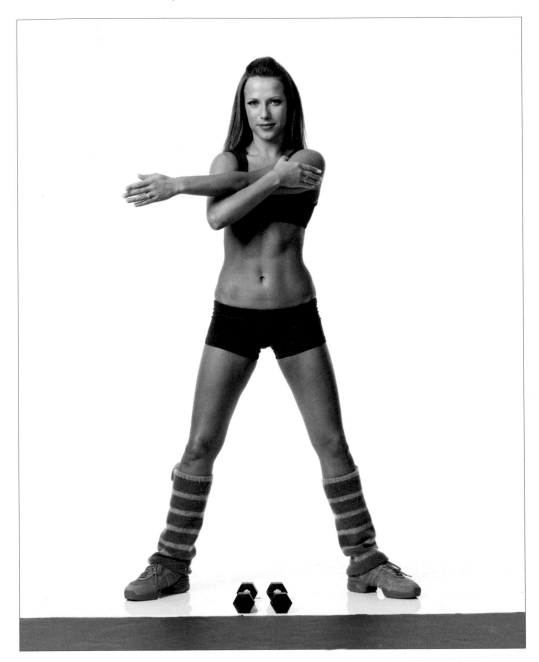

Extend one arm over the chest and across the body. Use the hand of the other arm to gently press against the extended arm, thereby giving the shoulder a relaxing stretch.

the dancer's abs and core

THE TERMS "core" and "stabilization" have become an integral part of the terminology of fitness instructors and personal trainers. Dance teachers, dancers, and choreographers have been familiar with both terms for decades.

In dance, the core represents much more than a group of muscles. It's the body's perceived center of energy. It's the area from which all movement emanates and from which all movements are controlled.

The core consists of a group of six abdominal muscles that form a layered, protective band around the spine and the rib cage, connecting both to the pelvis. The primary role of these muscles is postural—aiding in the maintenance of the upright stance. They're also involved in the process of breathing. The deepest of the core muscles—the transversus abdominis—is the closest to the spine and the most involved in keeping proper dance form and body alignment.

Just about all of the body's six-hundred and some muscles work in synchronized groups. In fact, it is physically and anatomically impossible to target just one specific muscle. For example, when you bend forward at the waist, the rectus abdominis (the so-called six-pack muscle) shortens while another group of muscles on your back extends. When you stand on one leg and raise the other, one group of front abdominal muscles is contracting to keep your leg extended, while a group of back muscles is also contracting to keep your spine stabilized.

This dance pose looks easy. But without Edyta's and Alec's firm ab muscles, she would not be able to sustain such a graceful arched back nor would he be able to counteract her line with such a strong stance.

When you command your elbow to bend, the biceps muscle shortens. It becomes an agonist muscle. But it is the triceps that, by extending, is stabilizing the upper arm and the shoulder, thus acting like an antagonist muscle.

Latin and rhythm dances require performers to frequently alternate between spinal flexing and stretching moves in all directions, so the dancers are constantly giving their core muscles a great workout. However, even when a day is filled with hours of dance practice, rehearsal and performance time—like the days of

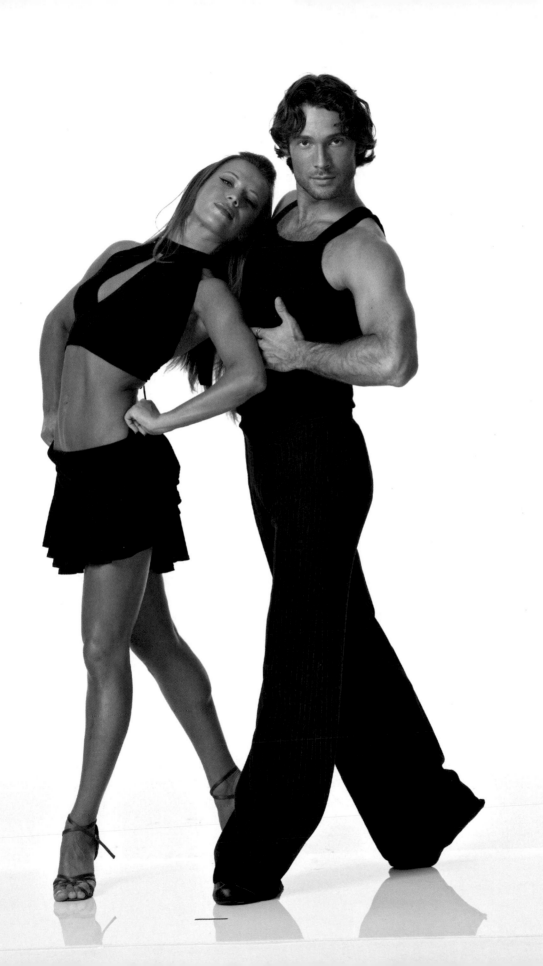

the dancer's abs and core

the professional and star contestants on *Dancing with the Stars*—many find a little extra time for a focused core workout.

Some people, especially men, spend a tremendous amount of time working the abs with the objective of that "six-pack" ab look. Unfortunately, doing hundreds of crunches and sit-ups does not guarantee that look. Diet and genetics also seem to play a major role. In addition, a superficial sculpted look—the result of the rectus abdominis muscle—does not necessarily equal a strong core.

If a dancer's firm waistline is something you'd like to aim for, then try a well-balanced diet, a regular workout schedule that includes cardiovascular exercise like the one in the *Cardio Dance* DVD, and the dance-based core exercises that follow.

Try doing the Standing Core Firmers five to six days a week. They will take only a few minutes of your time and you can do them just about anywhere. Then, two to three times a week, try the Mat Core Sequence. I don't promise that you'll end with a core as glamorously sculpted as Edyta's, but I guarantee that you will be very pleased with the changes you will see.

On the other hand, if you have not kept up with a regular exercise schedule that includes abdominal-strengthening exercises, or if you've ever had any muscular or skeletal spinal injury or back-related pain, you should consult with your general physician, chiropractor, or orthopedic surgeon before doing the exercises in this book or any abdominal exercise that's not supervised by a fitness expert.

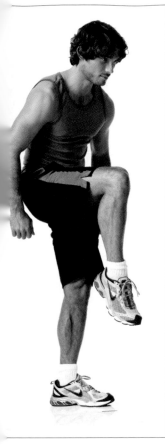

standing core firmers

exercise 1: standing curls

This exercise targets and engages the core muscles from various angles.

Starting position: Stand tall and with feet close together. Let the arms hang loosely along the sides of the body.

First Movement:

◀ *As you bring one knee toward the chest, bend forward over the thigh of the bent knee. Keeping the knee of your supporting leg slightly bent too will help your balance. However, overall balance depends on the strength and engagement of the core muscles.*

Second Movement:

▶ *1. This is a little more challenging all around, as you need to execute two movements at the same time while standing and balancing on one leg. At first, you might want to have a chair next to you for additional balance support. But what will really challenge the core muscles, the buttock muscles, and the hamstring muscles is performing this exercise repeatedly without any help.*

2. Extend the bent leg forward with its corresponding foot in a flexed position.

3. Now, straighten your back and stand tall. You do not need to extend the leg at hip level as Alec does, although that should be your ultimate target. The main objective here is core engagement and stabilization, not leg-extension height.

4. Bring the extended leg down to starting position, shift weight and do with the other leg.

Alternate between right and left for six to eight reps each. Don't rush this exercise. The slower you do this the more results you'll get.

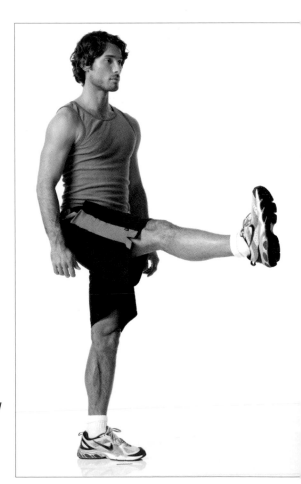

the dancer's abs and core

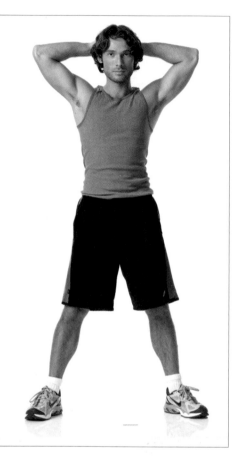

exercise 2: oblique crunches

This version of a standard mat exercise really helps to trim and tone the waistline area.

Starting position: Stand with feet wide apart. Place both hands behind your head with your elbows pointing sideways.

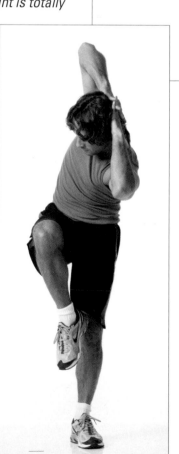

▶ *1. Shift your weight over to one leg, bring the knee of your free leg up to your chest while trying to meet it with the elbow of the opposite side of the body. Notice how Alec's weight is totally balanced in a straight line over the supporting foot and how his arms have stayed in one line.*

▶ *2. Bring the knee down, returning to starting position, and repeat the exercise with the other leg and elbow.*

Alternate between right and left for ten to twelve reps on each side.

mat core exercises

The core exercises featured in this portion of the book get progressively more intense. Unlike standard curls and crunches that are to be repeated countless times, the exercises here are to be done slowly and always with the best body alignment and form possible. None of them call for multiple repetitions. Quality over quantity!

A thin rubber mat, like a yoga or Pilates mat, is recommended. Heavily padded mats are not.

Proper breathing is important during any type of exercise, but more so during core exercises because the abdominal muscles are deeply involved in the function of the diaphragm during inhaling and exhaling. That's the reason for the emphasis on when to inhale and exhale during the following core exercises.

exercise 1: reverse curl

This is possibly the simplest of all abdominal exercises. You can learn a lot from it, though, about your own level of abdominal strength.

Starting position: Sit on your mat with your legs extended in front of you. Keep your knees bent and your legs and feet close together. Your torso should stand tall with shoulders down and arms extended downward alongside your body. Take a deep breath.

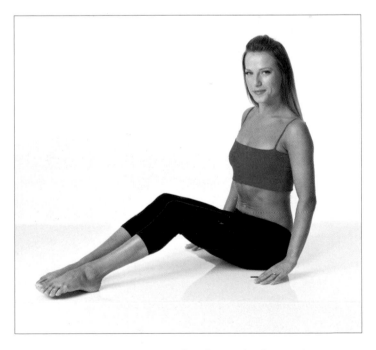

the dancer's abs and core

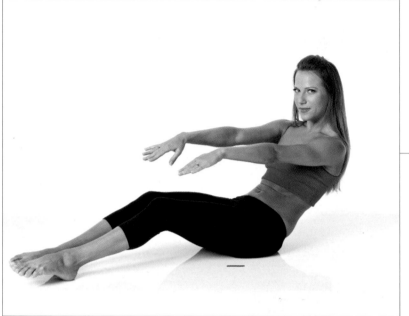

◀ *1. Exhale as you extend your arms forward and start to lean back toward the floor.*

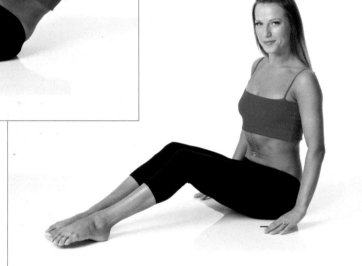

▶ *2. Inhale as you come back to your starting position.*

Four to eight Reverse Curls.

Correct Execution Tips

The feeling you should get right at the outset of this exercise is one of reaching forward with your fingertips as your tailbone tucks under and the backward rolling motion continues. You should also feel your lower abdominal muscles tightening during this rolling motion as they react against the pull of gravity. There's no need for you to roll back very far. In fact, if you focus on the progressively increasing contraction of your lower abs, you will sense what your reverse-curling limit is. Another way to sense your limit is when you feel the heels of your feet starting to come off the floor. That means that your thigh muscles—adductors and abductors alike—have come in to rescue you. Remember, you want to work the core. We'll take care of the thighs in another exercise sequence.

exercise 2: half curls

This exercise brings the thigh and the core muscles into play.

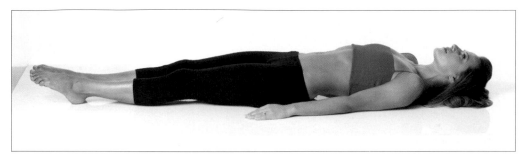

Starting position: Lie back on the mat with your body fully extended and arms at your sides. Take a deep breath.

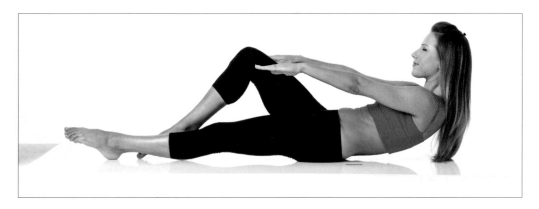

As you exhale, you need to do the following:
1. Bring your chin into your chest.
2. Firm your abs as you lift your shoulders off the mat.
3. Bring one knee toward your curling torso.
4. Continue reaching forward.
5. Keep the other leg fully extended with its toes pointed. Slowly roll back to the starting position. As you roll back, think of placing one vertebra at a time on the mat.

Inhale and repeat with the other leg.   **Four reps on each leg.**

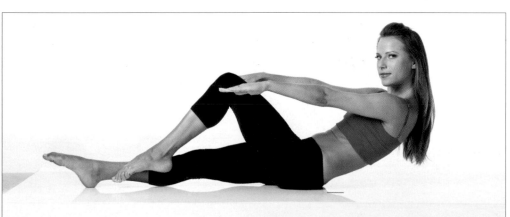

the dancer's abs and core

exercise 3: scissors

This exercise is one of the best waistline chiselers there is. It does take a little practice. It also demands full engagement of the core muscles.

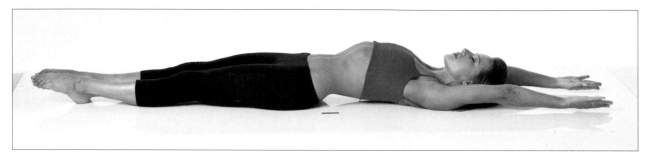

Starting position: Lie on the mat with your body fully extended.

▶ *1. Bring one leg straight up toward your torso as you curl the torso toward that leg. Place your hands behind the leg just under the knee and give the leg a gentle stretch toward your chest. Release the leg and the hold, but keep your shoulders off the mat.*

▶ *2. Bring the other leg up.*

Alternate between right and left leg for ten to twelve reps.

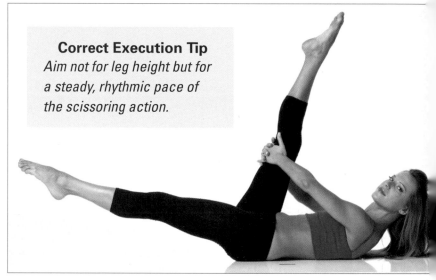

Correct Execution Tip
Aim not for leg height but for a steady, rhythmic pace of the scissoring action.

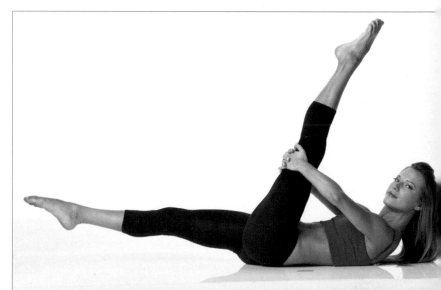

exercise 4: advance oblique toners

The external oblique muscles, one of the six muscle groups of the core, wrap around the body between the rib cage and the front edge of the hips. Not only does this muscle group work hard during the torso-twisting and hip-grinding movements characteristic of Latin dances, but it is the muscle group most responsible for that sculpted, pinned-in, waistline and for that curvaceous hip look.

Correct Execution Tips
Keep your lower back well stabilized by pressing your abs against the lower spine. You should also keep your upper torso stabilized by pressing your arms down against the mat.

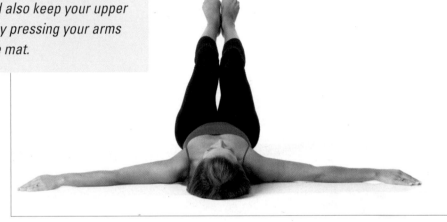

Starting position: Lie back on the mat with arms extended sideways and knees bent over the lower abs. Inhale deeply.

▶ *1. Extend both legs straight up and slightly to one side of the body.*

2. Exhale, then inhale as you bring the knees back down to the starting position.

3. Exhale again as you then extend the legs to the other side.

Six to ten reps on each side.

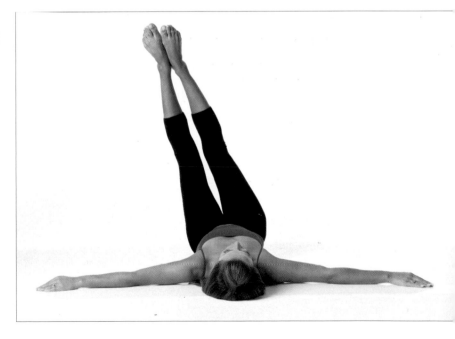

the dancer's abs and core

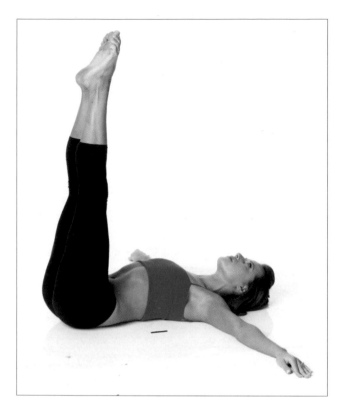

exercise 5: reverse leg lifts

There are many ways to do leg lifts, all of which engage the core muscles to an extent. This one calls for lowering the legs from a ninety-degree vertical starting position to no less than a forty-five degree angle off the floor.

▶ *1. Keep the legs fully extended and the feet pointing. Inhale.*

▶ *2. Flex both feet and lower the legs. Exhale, then inhale, bringing the legs back up to their vertical starting position.*

Four to six reps.

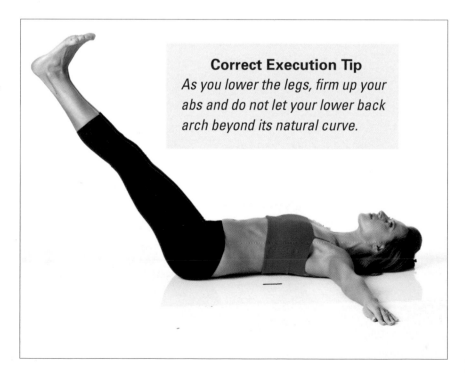

Correct Execution Tip
As you lower the legs, firm up your abs and do not let your lower back arch beyond its natural curve.

exercise 6: moderate v-sit

There are many versions of this exercise. The one that follows is a moderately intensive one.

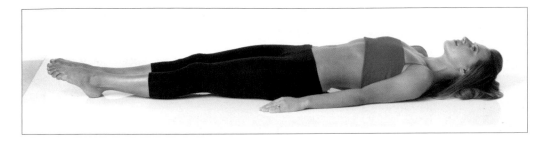

1. Lie back on the mat with your body fully extended and arms placed by your sides. Inhale.

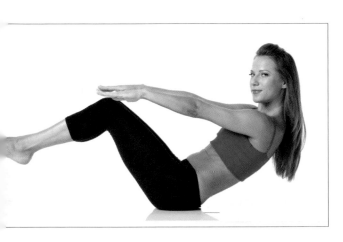

◀ *2. Exhale as you fold the body in half by bending the knees toward the chest and lifting your back off the mat. For added balance, extend the arms forward toward the knee. Your objective should be to keep your chest up and your back straight. Your folded body will be forming the shape of a "V".*

Correct Execution Tips

Feel well balanced on the Half-V-Sit position before extending the legs to the full V-Sit. When reaching the full V-Sit position, you should feel as if your legs and your torso are in a constant upward stretching mode. The higher you extend your legs, the closer your torso should be to them.

▶ *3. Extend your legs up and out. This is the full V-Sit position. Keep your shoulders down, your arms extended, and your torso feeling tall and elongated. Inhale.*

4. Return to Half-V-Sit position.

5. Exhale as you roll slowly back down to your starting position.

Four reps.

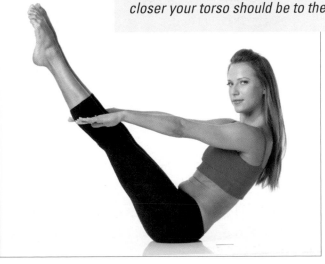

the dancer's abs and core

exercise 7: v-sit challenger

Once you feel confident and strong doing the Moderate V-Sit, give yourself a challenge. Here's how.

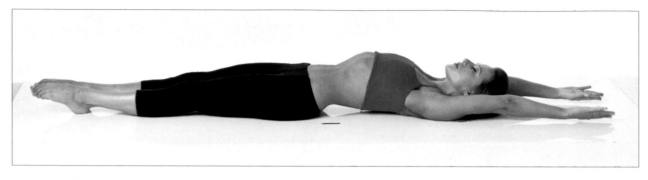

1. Lie on the mat with the body fully extended from the fingertips to the tips of the toes. Inhale.

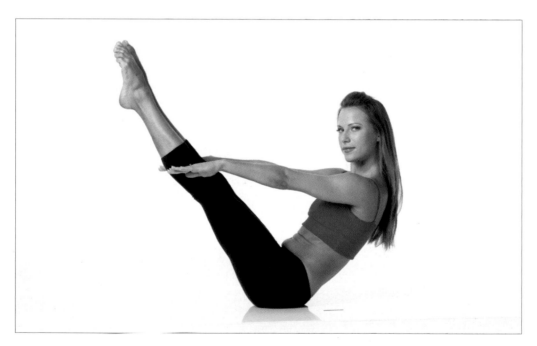

2. Exhale as you aim for the full V-Sit in one controlled move. Inhale as you return to the fully extended position.

exercise 8: the plank

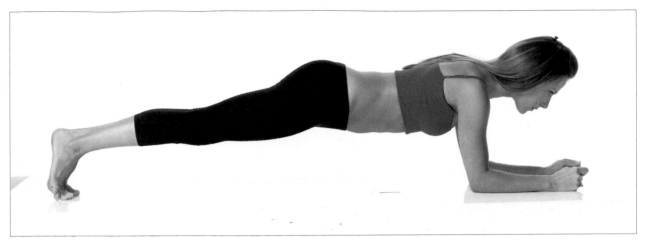

This very simple exercise requires little other than holding what's called a Plank position for twenty to thirty seconds. Core muscles must be kept firmly held as the body is being balanced between the toes and the elbows. The spine needs to be kept long and maintain its natural curve. Notice that the neck is also held long and horizontal, parallel to the floor.

exercise 9: child's pose

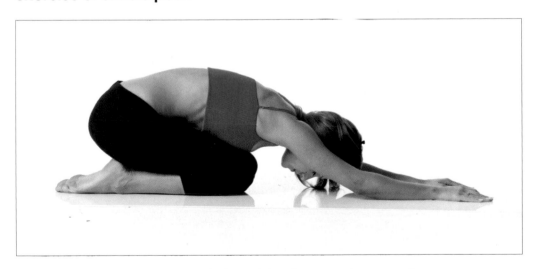

Little feels as good as this stretch done right after a good core workout.

paso doble thighs, buns, and hips

IN ADDITION TO THE PASO DOBLE, the *Dancing With the Stars Cardio Dance* DVD also features the Cha-cha and the Samba. In dance competitions, all three dances are grouped under the Latin division. However, the Cha-cha is of Cuban origin, Paso Doble is Spanish, and the Samba is Brazilian.

Characteristically, the signature dance patterns of the Samba and the Cha-cha consist of short sequences of individual steps danced to a syncopated rhythm. Maintaining body contact is not a technical requirement of these dances; this allows dancers to change into and out of various apart dance positions. It also allows dancers more freedom of choreography.

Latin dance music is all about beating drums and shaking maracas. It lends itself to lots of theatrical, isolated movements of the shoulders, rib cage, and hips, which dancers can execute as fast as a finger snap or sensuously slow. While strong core muscles are key in the control and speed of dance isolations, the strength and firmness of the hip, thigh, and buttock muscles are just as important.

The muscles of the buttocks, hips, and thighs are functionally interrelated. Therefore, most exercises for the hips and buttocks employ the legs as levers that repeatedly engage the muscles in those two areas. In other exercises we need to place our bodies in positions that use the pull of gravity to help further target those areas. Not only can the muscles of these three major areas sustain a tough workout, they practically require it.

The exercises that follow combine standard strength-training exercises with dance-based moves that are themselves qualify as muscle-strengthening moves.

matador's thighs

The Paso Doble features lots of lunges, knee drops, and crawls, and dramatic "picture poses." All of these call for strong thigh muscles. But strong thighs need not be bulky ones. They need to be functionally strong—able to sustain the body's weight on one extended leg or on a bent knee, and then to spring it back up in a split second. Fortunately, one doesn't need to do a lot of different exercises to really strengthen the thighs, knees, and buttocks. A few good ones are all you need.

The following exercises are challenging and effective. They will tax your strength, your balance, and your coordination. If you know you have weak knees or if you've had any sort of knee- or hip-related problem, you should consult with your doctor before trying any of these exercises. Once you're given the OK, you might want to use a chair for additional balance and stability support. You might also want to have a workout partner or a certified fitness instructor to spot your body form and execution while you do these exercises.

exercise 1: crunch squats

Squats are one of the greatest thigh and buttock firmers, and this version is a real burner. The emphasis here is not on the squat itself but on the push-off into a vertical crunch position from a squat position.

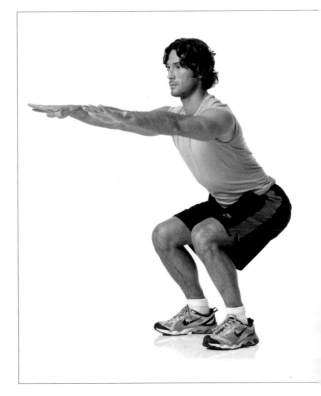

The push-off action and the simultaneous weight change work the thighs and the buttocks. Standing on one leg further activates the core muscles to stabilize you, as well as working the hip and thigh muscles of the leg you're standing on. The forward leaning action into a bent leg also activates the core muscles.

▶ Starting position: Start from a squat position: Feet are parallel to each other and shoulder-width apart. Knees are directly over the toes. Arms are fully extended in front of the body, and ab muscles are firmly held.

paso doble thighs, buns, and hips

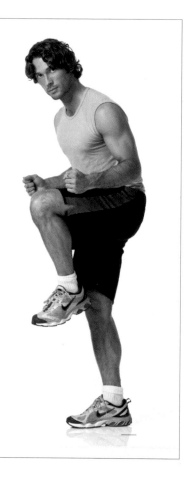

Three different movements need to take place at the same time as you push off into a standing position:

◀ 1. As you push off to a standing position, let your body's weight shift to one leg.

2. As you center and balance your weight on the one standing leg, bring the knee of the other leg toward your chest.

3. As you bend that knee, curl your arms and let your torso lean toward the bent leg, keeping your back as long as possible.

▶ Return to your starting position.

Repeat steps 1–3 on the other leg.

Eight to twelve reps on each leg.

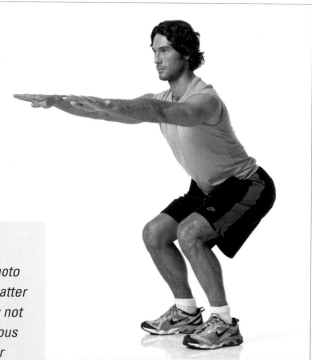

Correct Execution Tip

Do you see the difference between the previous photo of Alec's Crunch Squat and the photo here? In the latter photo, Alec's knees are not as bent, and his body is not sitting as low. This is a more moderate, less strenuous squat. Undoubtedly, the lower you squat, the harder the buttock and hip muscles have to contract to get you back up. However, when you first try this exercise, starting with a moderate-level squat will help you focus on your coordination and balance a lot more easily.

exercise 2: crunch lunges

This exercise is quite similar to the previous one, but instead of starting from a squat position you start from a lunge position, and you do not alternate legs in the same set.

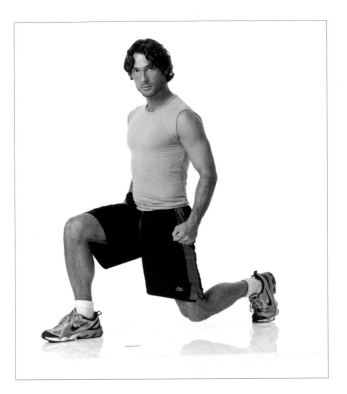

◀ Starting position: Step back into a lunge position. Your aim is to balance your body's weight equally between your front leg and back leg. The front knee should be directly over its corresponding foot. The angle of the bent knee should never exceed ninety degrees. The torso should be kept upright and the core muscles firm. Let your arms rest alongside your body.

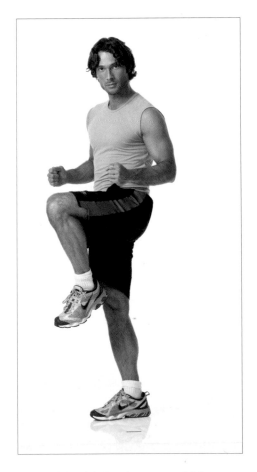

As during Exercise 1, three different movements need to take place at the same time that you push off into a standing position:

▶ *1. Push off to a standing position on one leg.*

2. Bring your non-weight-bearing knee toward your chest.

3. Curl your arms as you lean forward toward the bent knee. Return to your standing position.

Six to ten reps on each leg.

paso doble thighs, buns, and hips

exercise 3: contra-body progressive lunges

Admittedly, this is a challenging exercise that consists of two alternating forward lunges—one on each leg—followed by two alternating back lunges. What makes this short sequence a little more intense is twisting the entire torso in opposition to the lunging leg. This means if you are lunging forward with the right leg, you need to twist the torso to the right so as to bring your left shoulder toward the right knee. In dance, the moving of the upper body in opposition to the moving leg is referred to as contra-body movement. This exercise sequence really taxes your strength, balance, and endurance.

Starting Position: Stand tall with elbows bent and placed along side the body. Keep your weight on your left foot.

1. Lunge forward with the right leg, twisting the upper body to the right. (This is a contra-body lunge.)

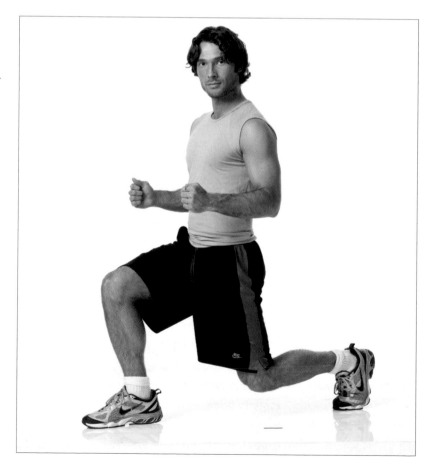

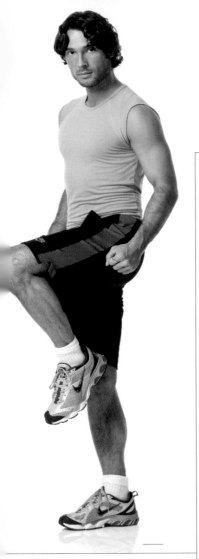

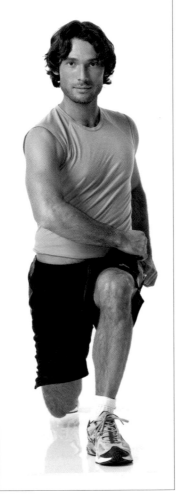

◀ 2. Standing on the right leg, bring the left knee up into a vertical crunch.

◀ 3. Lunge forward with the left leg, twisting the upper body to the left.

4. Standing on the left leg, bring the right knee up into a vertical crunch.

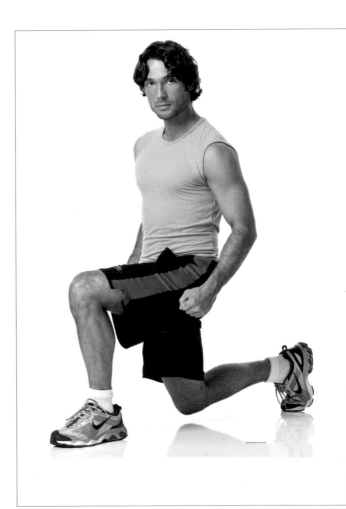

Repeat this sequence of two forward contra-body lunges and two back contra-body lunges a few times. Keep tabs on how many you do during each workout. It's a great way to track how much stronger your thighs and buttocks are getting.

▶ 5. Lunge back with the right leg, twisting the upper body to the left.

6. Follow with a vertical crunch, standing on the right leg.

7. Follow with a contra-body lunge, moving back with the left leg.

8. Follow with another vertical crunch, standing on the left leg.

paso doble thighs, buns, and hips

exercise 4: matador's lunge

This exercise combines a characteristic Paso Doble lunge pose with a standing bullfighter's pose that's also a wonderful stretch for the chest and shoulders.

◀ Starting position: Stand tall with feet together. Raise the right arm high with the palm of the hand turned in toward the body and its shoulder leaning back. Feel the stretch on the shoulder and chest muscles.

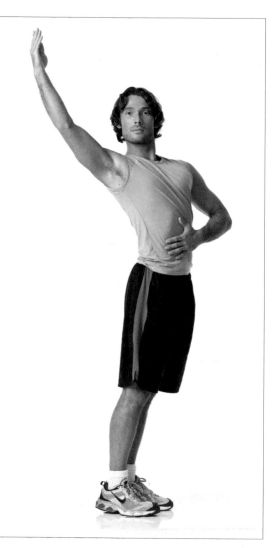

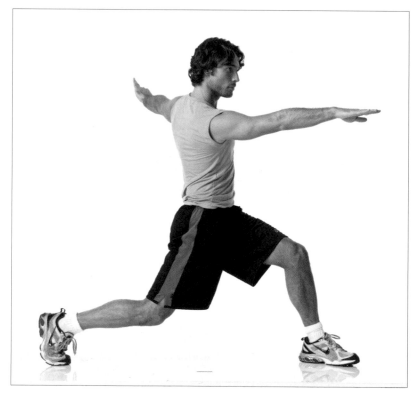

▶ 1. Lunge to the left. Twist the upper body toward the lunging leg. Extend the right arm forward in the direction of the left leg. Extend the left arm out to the side.

2. Use your thigh muscles to push yourself back up into the matador-stretch starting position.

Six to eight lunges to each side.
If no one is looking, immediately after your last stretch, you are allowed to yell out "Olé!"

amazing buns and hips

exercise 1: front vertical pumps

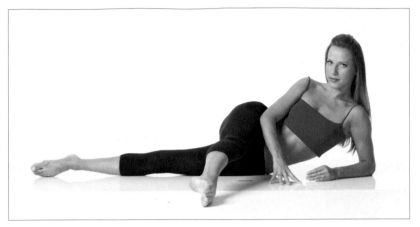

◀ Starting position: Lie on one side. Extend one leg forward at hip level. The top leg should be turned slightly inward from the hip.

1. Use one elbow to support your torso and to keep it tall and extended. Bring the other arm across the front of your body, placing the hand on the mat. This position will help you from rolling forward too much.

◀ *2. Lift the extended leg about two feet up from the floor.*

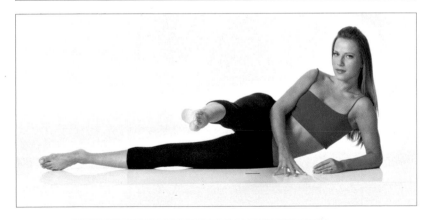

◀ *3. Lower the leg to about one foot from the floor. Continue lifting and lowering the leg between those two heights as if it were a water pump.*

Fifteen to twenty repetitions on both sides.

> **Correct Execution Tip**
> *It is important that the hip socket closest to the floor is in a direct vertical line with the hip socket above it.*

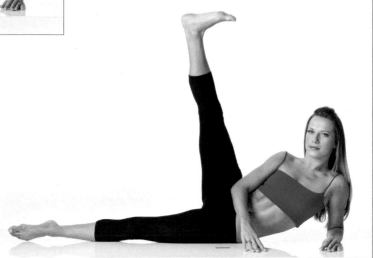

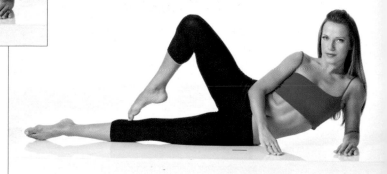

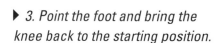

paso doble thighs, buns, and hips

exercise 2:
hip flexion and contraction

◀ Starting position: Lying on one side, bend the top knee and point it straight up. Point the foot as well. Hip sockets should remain vertically aligned.

▶ *1. With the foot flexed, extend the leg up. Feel the muscles of the leg being engaged all the way from the hip socket to the Achilles tendon, where the calf meets the foot.*

◀ *2. With the foot still flexed, bring the leg down slowly to meet the other leg.*

▶ *3. Point the foot and bring the knee back to the starting position.*

Ten to twelve reps on each side.

exercise 3a: forward and back extensions

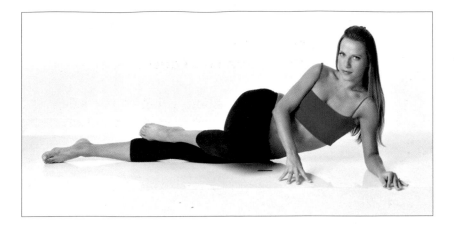

◀ Starting position: Lie on one side with the top knee bent

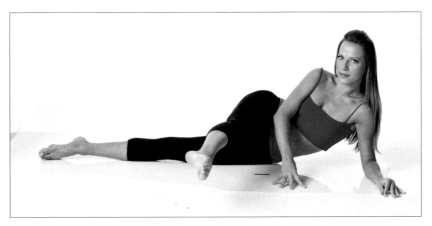

◀ *1. Extend the leg forward. Keep the abs firm and also keep the side of the body closest to the floor long and stable.*

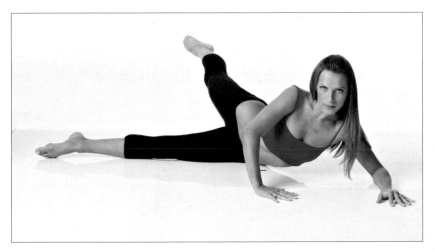

◀ *2. Swing the extended leg backward. Let the top of the body lean slightly forward as the leg is at its farthest back point.*

3. Bend the knee of the extended leg, moving it to the starting position, ready for it to be extended forward again.

Ten to twelve forward and back extensions followed by Exercise 3B.

paso doble thighs, buns, and hips

exercise 3b: reverse hip pumps

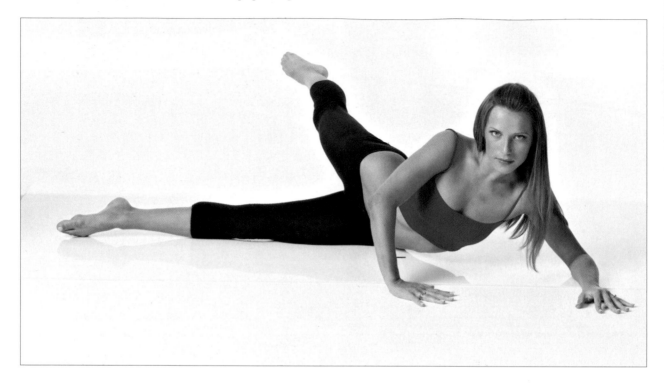

1. Lean forward and extend the leg behind you.

2. Tap the floor with the toes and immediately raise the leg to about two feet off the ground. Do not let the upper hip roll back.

3. Bring the leg down again, tapping the floor with the toes.

Fifteen to twenty repetitions, then switch sides and start with Exercise 3A using the other leg.

exercise 4a: bun crunchers a

This exercise calls for a thigh action resembling that of an old water pump. However the objective of Bun Crunchers A and B is not as much to keep pumping the leg up and down as it is to maintain the good old gluteus maximus in a state of contraction for a long period of time. You'll know just how long that period should be!

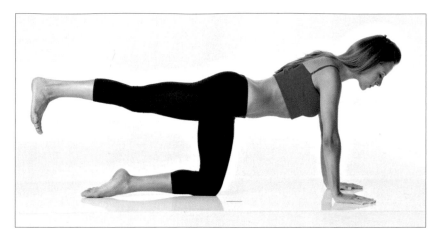

◀ Starting position: Begin facedown, on your hands and one knee, supporting and balancing your body between the arms and knee. Extend the thigh of the non-weight-bearing leg to a position that's parallel to the floor.

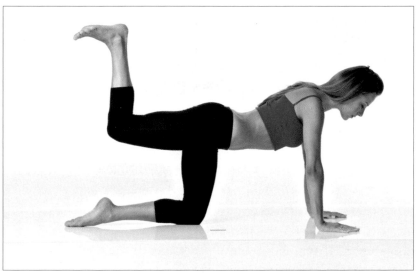

◀ *1. Bend the knee of the extended leg and flex its foot. Keep the core muscles firm.*

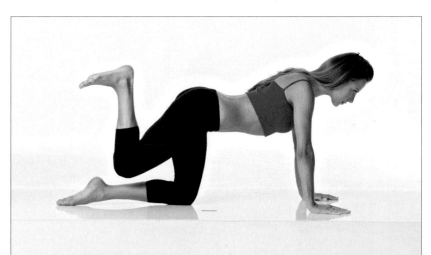

◀ *2. Bring the bent knee down toward the floor then raise the leg back up to the starting position.*

Ten to twelve reps, followed by Bun Crunchers B.

217

paso doble thighs, buns, and hips

exercise 4b: bun crunchers b

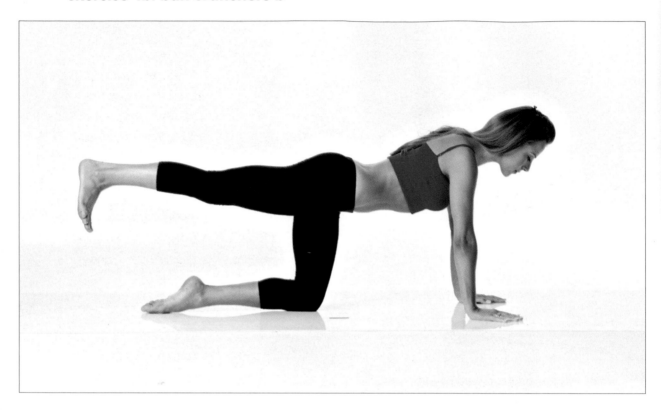

Starting Position: Begin facedown, on your hands and one knee, supporting and balancing your body between the arms and knee. Extend the thigh of the non-weight-bearing leg to a position that's parallel to the floor. Then, raise and lower the thigh as if it were a pump. Make sure to also keep the entire pelvic structure horizontal. The tendency during this movement is for the pelvis to move. It should remain stabilized through firm core engagement.

exercise 5: the burning bridge

If you've never heard the term "feel the burn," you will soon be very familiar with its meaning.

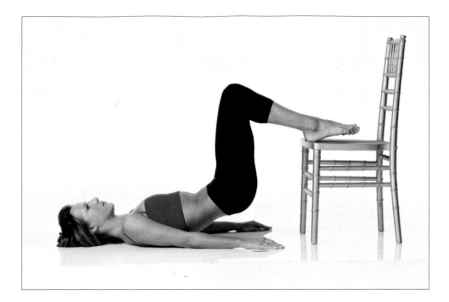

◀ Starting Position: Place your heels on the seat of a chair. Make sure this chair is propped against a wall or against a heavy piece of furniture that won't allow the chair to slide. Bring your buttocks as close to the edge of the chair's seat as possible. And let both arms rest alongside your body.

▶ *1. Tightening the buttocks and pressing down on the seat of the chair with your feet, bring your lower body up until you form an imaginary straight line that starts at the base of the shoulders and ends at the knees.*

2. Lower your body a couple of feet.

3. Then press down on your feet again, contracting the buttocks and core muscles and lifting the body back up to a bridge position. This movement should be performed slowly.

Continue the elevating and lowering of the body until you feel that your buttock muscles are starting to fatigue (that's the burn!). But don't stop there. See if you can burn through five or six more reps.

jive dancing: quick feet and great legs

THE SWING is America's own native dance. There are two basic styles of the American Swing. One is called the East Coast Swing, also referred to as the Triple Swing, and the other is called the West Coast Swing. Both styles share roots dating back to musical and dance styles of the Roaring Twenties: ragtime, blues, jazz, the Shag, the Lindy Hop, the Charleston.

The Jive is a faster-paced version of the American Swing.

For competition dancers, the Jive is a choreographic challenge. In addition to the variety of tunes and rhythmic changes the Jive can be performed to, dancers have a virtually unlimited repertoire of dance movements that are symbolic of bygone eras to choose from for their routines; they range from basic soft-shoe and Charleston dance sequences to acrobatic moves like cartwheels, straddle jumps, splits, and just about anything their minds can make their legs and feet do—and do quickly.

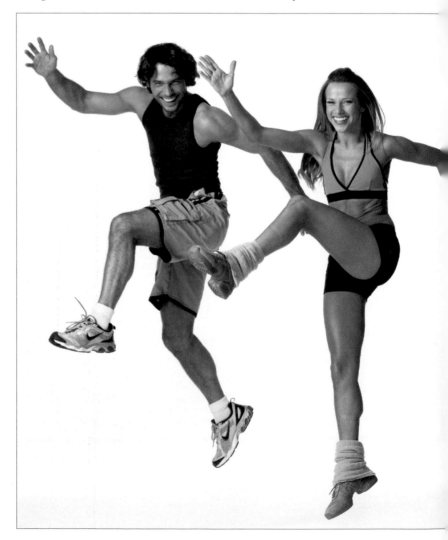

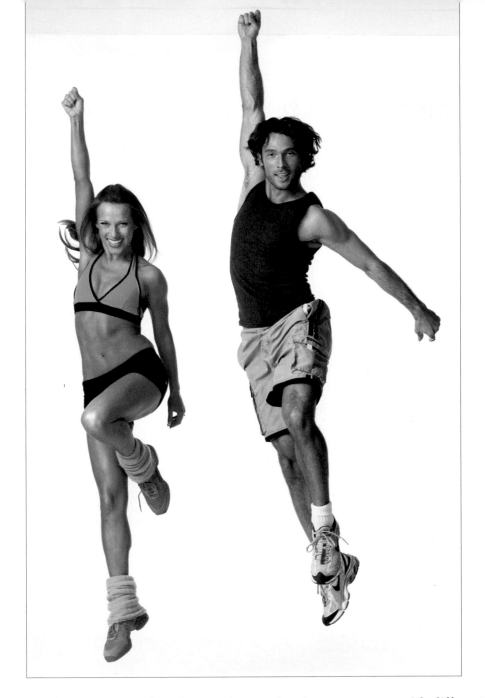

While putting together Jive routines and trying to come up with different dance moves, many dance teams have been known to act and play a little like kids, as this photo sequence of Alec and Edyta proves.

Dancing a basic Swing or Jive is within nearly anyone's reach in a very short period of time. Adding jumps, kicks, swivels, fast turns, and amazing splits to a dance routine take lots of training and practice time. It also takes strong legs, ankles, and feet. The following exercises will help you strengthen yours.

jive dancing: quick feet and great legs

exercise 1: first-position ankle and calf toners

For this exercise, you might first use a chair for better balance and body alignment. You could also stand next to a wall for support. However, doing these exercises without the assistance of a chair or wall will force you to use the core muscles that much more.

Starting position: Stand tall with legs and feet turned out. In ballet, this position is referred to as the "first position of the feet," and the bending of the knees you are about to perform is called a "plié."

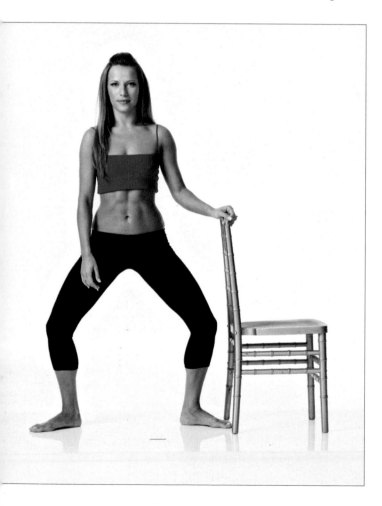

◀ *1. Bend your knees in the direction of your toes without letting your pelvis tilt backward.*

2. Keep your body's weight grounded in the center of each foot.

3. When you feel the heels of your feet starting to come off the floor, you should stop bending.

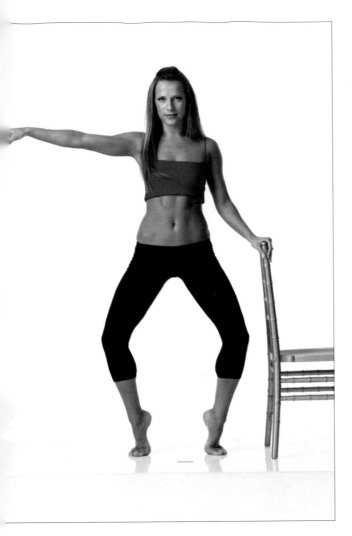

4. Keeping the knees firmly placed over the toes, raise the heels of both feet until you are standing on the balls of your feet. The objective here is to not allow the rest of your body to rise as the heels rise. This strengthens both the feet and the calf muscles.

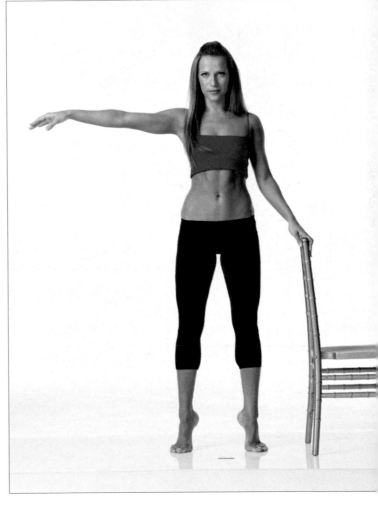

5. Press the balls of your feet against the floor and straighten your legs. You should feel the inner and outer muscles of your thighs contracting.

6. Now, reverse the movement. Bend your knees again, but keep your weight balanced on the balls of your feet.

Repeat this sequence two to four times. This is also a great exercise for strengthening the arches of the feet, especially if you increase your reps to six to eight times.

jive dancing: quick feet and great legs

exercise 2: second-position ankle and calf toners

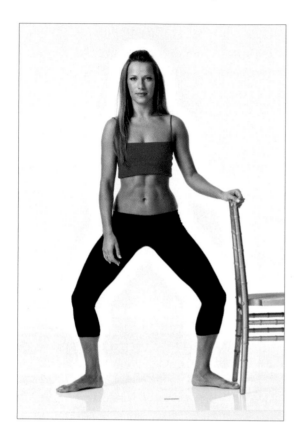

This exercise sequence follows the same process as Exercise 1. However, it is a slightly more challenging, more intense toner of the feet and of the inner and outer thighs.

◀ *1. Do a second-position plié as pictured.*

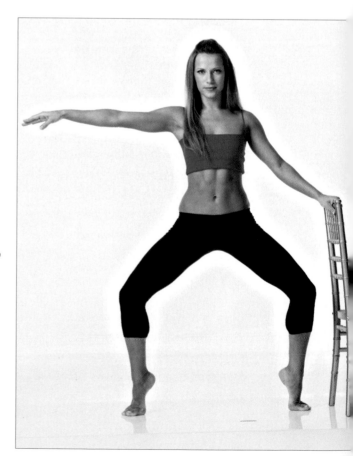

▶ *2. Lift the heels of the feet without letting the entire body rise. Make sure that each knee is moving directly over the toes.*

3. Press down on the toes, straightening the knees and the legs. Feel tall and long.

4. Reverse the movement as in Exercise 1.

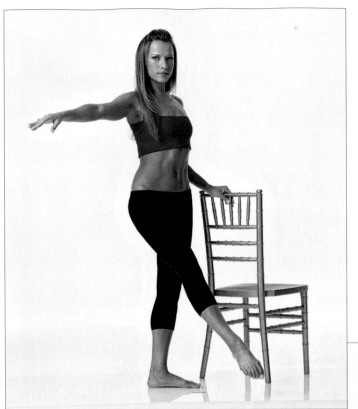

exercise 3: toe flexion and extension

This is a very simple, feel-so-good movement that actually involves all the major muscles and tendons of the legs and the feet.

◀ *Stand on one leg with the other leg extended forward and the foot pointed.*

▶ *Flex the foot. The objective of this movement goes beyond the obvious flexing of the foot: The main objective is to feel the calf muscle elongating as the foot flexes.*

Point and flex eight to ten times. Then change feet. Your feet and legs should now be well warmed up for the following exercise sequence.

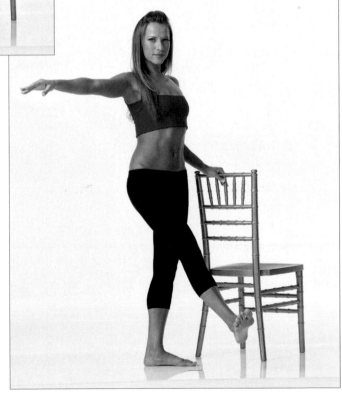

jive dancing: quick feet and great legs

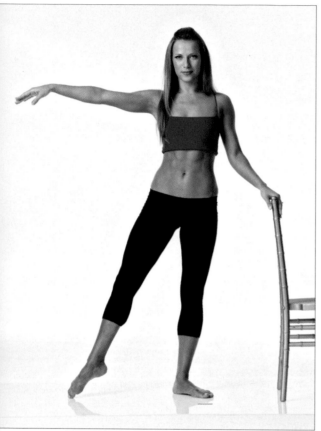

exercise 4: lateral extension

Focused, slow Lateral Extensions strengthen leg muscles and increase their hip-socket range of motion.

◀ Starting Position: Stand on a turned-out leg while the free leg is extended sideways with a pointed foot.

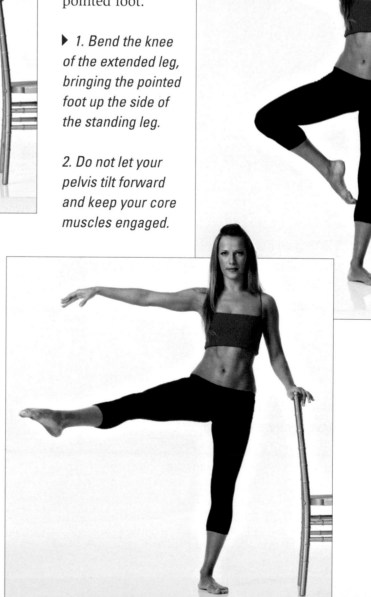

▶ *1. Bend the knee of the extended leg, bringing the pointed foot up the side of the standing leg.*

2. Do not let your pelvis tilt forward and keep your core muscles engaged.

▶ *3. Keeping the knee stabilized, extend the leg outward with a pointed foot.*

4. Lower the extended leg back down to your starting position and repeat the sequence.

Six to eight lateral extensions on each side.

exercise 5: front extension

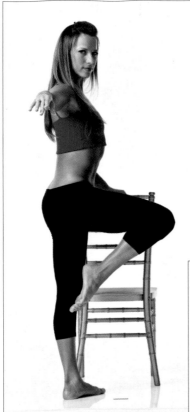

Starting Position: Stand with feet together, parallel to each other.

◀ *1. Bend one knee, keeping it pointed straight in front of you.*

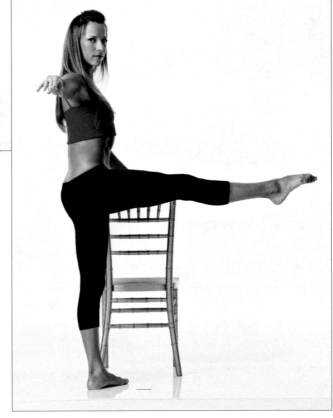

▶ *2. Extend the leg forward, keeping the supporting leg straight and the core muscles firm.*

3. Bring the leg back to its bent-knee starting position.

Six to eight front extensions on each leg.

jive dancing: quick feet and great legs

exercise 6: arabesque toners a and b

The mechanics of this exercise are simple. However, its effectiveness largely depends on correct body posture and alignment.

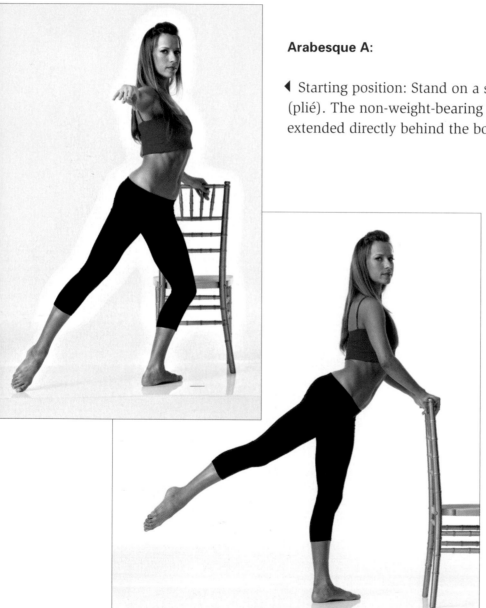

Arabesque A:

◀ Starting position: Stand on a slightly bent knee (plié). The non-weight-bearing leg should be extended directly behind the body.

◀ *As you straighten your supporting leg, lift the extended leg to the height of your supporting knee or higher. The top of the pointed foot and front of the knee should be facing the floor. As you lift, keep your core muscles firm and let your upper torso lean slightly forward. The body pose that results from this dance movement is referred to as an Arabesque.*

Six to eight reps. Then follow with Arabesque B.

Arabesque B:

After your execute your last Arabesque lift, hold the leg in the Arabesque position. Then lower it a couple of inches and lift it back to the full Arabesque position. Pump the extended leg ten to fourteen times. The objective of this movement is to keep the buttocks muscles in a state of contraction until muscle fatigue sets in. Once you complete the reps for A and B, change to the other leg.

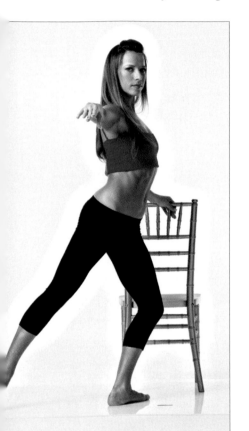

exercise 7:
jazz dance kicks

This type of leg kick works the buttocks and the thigh muscles.

◀ Starting position: Stand on a bent knee. Extend the other leg directly behind your body with the foot pointed.

▶ *1. Straighten the standing leg a little bit as you swing the free leg straight up.*

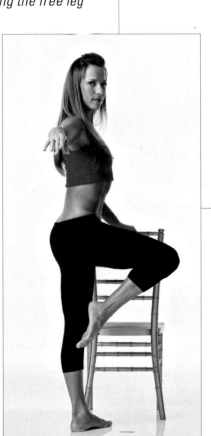

▶ *2. Instead of keeping the leg extended when you swing it back down, bend the knee. Stand tall on a straight supporting leg.*

3. Then, extend the leg back to its starting position as you bend your supporting leg.

Four to eight kicks on each side.

cool-down stretches

ALTHOUGH THE MAJORITY of our exercises are based on dynamic conditioning, meaning strengthening combined with stretching, every workout session should be followed by a stretching segment. The longer the workout segment, the longer the stretching segment should be.

The following exercises feature a series of passive stretches. Passive stretches are those where you place your body in a specific position that targets a specific muscle group, and then gradually aim for further overall relaxation in that position and for stretching the ligaments that connect muscles to bones. For more effectiveness, passive stretching should always be coordinated with a breathing pattern: slow inhalations and exhalations.

first stretch - standing back and hamstring stretch

Starting Position: Stand with feet apart and slightly turned out. Keep hips facing directly forward.

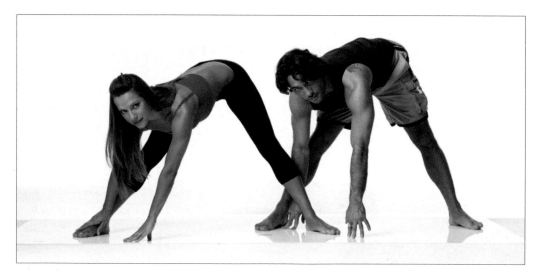

1. Turn your torso to the right about 45 degrees (or to the 1:00 o'clock mark).

2. Bend forward, keeping your back straight. Let your arms drop toward the floor. Do not bend over the front of your right thigh or beyond. The body should be kept toward the inside of your right leg.

3. Let your head drop.

4. Take a deep breath. Exhale and let your body bend further from the waist. You'll feel your hamstring muscles tightening and trying to resist your bending. That's ok.

5. Take another deep breath. Exhale and let your body relax further in that position.

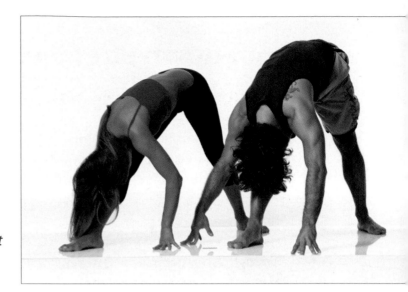

6. Take another breath. Exhale then roll back up, one vertebra at a time, to your starting position.

7. Switch sides by turning the torso to the left.

You don't need to switch from right to left. One good relaxing stretch on each side is plenty.

second stretch - inner thigh and groin stretch

Starting Position: Take a large lunge step to the side. The bending knee should be pointing in the same heel-to-toe straight line as its corresponding foot. The top of the body should be leaning forward. You can place your hands on the floor in front of your for support.

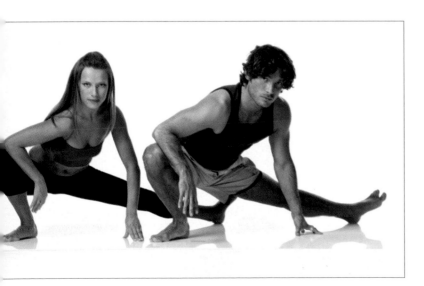

1. Take a deep breath. Exhale as you let your body go further down toward the floor. Flex the foot of the extended leg. Inhale.

2. Exhale and now let your body lean further forward. Stay in that position for a few seconds keeping up a slow and even breathing rhythmic pattern.

3. Switch sides.

cool-down stretches

third stretch - sitting hamstring and calf stretch

Starting Position: Sit on the floor with one leg extended diagonally out to the side. The other leg should be bent with its foot placed in front of the pelvis. You should be sitting on both "sits bones."

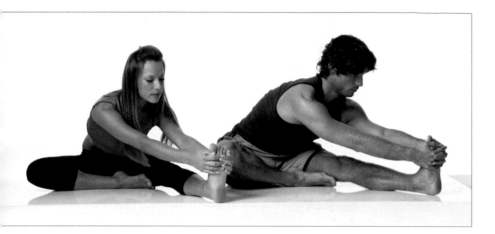

1. Lean forward over the extended leg. Keep that foot flexed. If you can reach your toes, clasp your hands around the ball of the foot. If not, clasp your hands around your ankle.

2. Inhale deeply. Exhale as you lean farther forward in the direction of your toe. Hold that position for at least 10 seconds. That is now your new starting position.

3. Inhale again then exhale and try to reach further forward a couple more inches. Then hold that position for at least 10 seconds.

Correct Execution Tips
The objective here is not to approach this movement as a forward bend. Instead, the objective is to keep as long a back as possible when going forward toward the foot.

Correct Execution Tips
Here again the more forward you lean, the tighter the back of the extended leg is going to feel until you relax everything in that position before stretching further.

You should also aim to keep the leg well extended. However, if you know your hamstrings are very tight, you can keep a slight bend on the extended knee.

4. Spend at least 3 or 4 minutes in this position before switching to the other side. And NEVER BOUNCE INTO A STRETCH. Take it slow and easy.

fourth stretch - total forward stretch

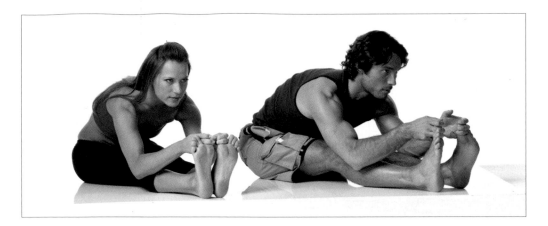

Starting Position: Sit with both legs extended forward and feet flexed. Bend your upper body over the top of the thighs and let your arms extend forward. You can either grab your toes or let your arms rest along side the calves.

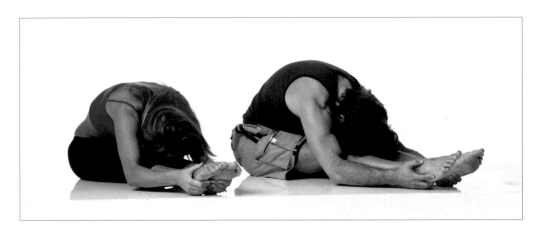

1. The same principle as for the last stretch applies here. Coordinate your breathing patterns with your stretching by taking a deep breath then stretching during the exhalation. This time try pointing the toes as you lean forward.

Correct Execution Tips
Unlike the previous stretch, you can let your back round as you lean forward. Focus not on how far forward you are reaching, but on giving the muscles enough time to adjust to the position in which you are stretching them before trying to stretch farther.

cool-down stretches

fifth stretch - straddle/second position stretch

Alec and Edyta have very flexible hips that allow both of them to straddle out in what in dance we refer to as a second position stretch. Do not let their flexibility intimidate you.

Starting Position: Sit on floor with legs extended outward and feet pointed. Your torso should be sitting tall and long. Lift your left arm straight up from the shoulder. Bring the other arm across your waistline and over to the opposite side of the body.

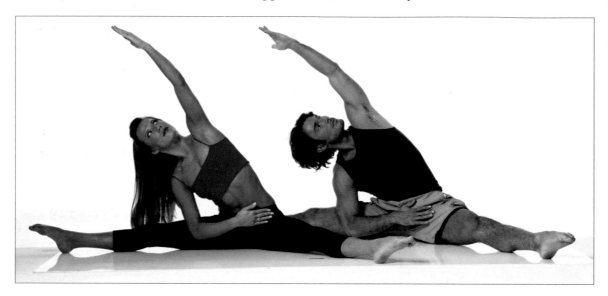

1. The simplest way to describe how to do this stretch would be "bend sideways to the right over the right leg." However, that is not exactly what you should think of doing while performing this move. Look at this photo of Alec and Edyta. What they are doing is elongating one side of their bodies (the left side) up and away from the extended leg (the left leg), while leaning toward their right leg. They are, in fact, stretching all the muscles that start from the tip of the toes of the left foot, the muscles of the leg and thigh, those of the sides of the body and right up to the tips of the fingers of the left hand.

Repeat the stretch on the opposite side.

2. As with previous stretches, breathe in when you reach a stretched position. Then stay in that position for a few seconds, breathing normally. Then take another deep breath, letting out the air slowly as you stretch further.

sixth stretch - hip stretch

Too few people do this stretch, although it is one that should be a part of any-one's regular workout routine. For dancers and athletes, especially fast-walkers or runners, this is an extremely important stretch.

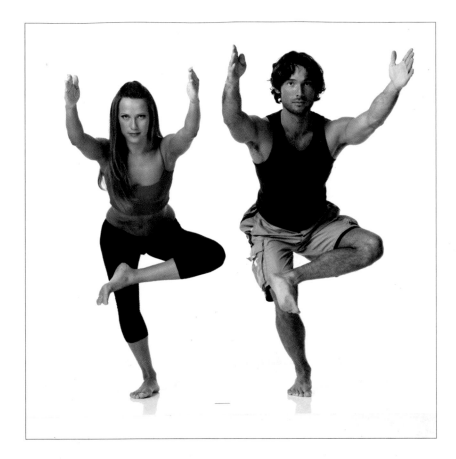

1. Stand on one leg, keeping the leg and foot slightly turned out from its hip socket.

2. Bend the knee of the other leg, placing its foot just above the knee of the standing leg.

3. Take a deep breath. Exhale as you bend the standing knee as well as lean forward at the waist. Reach up toward the ceiling with both arms, keeping your back as flat and long as possible. Keep that position for a few seconds.

4. Take another deep breath. Exhale. Sit back and reach up and forward further. Spend a few seconds in this position.

5. Switch to the other side and repeat all four steps.

Correct Execution Tip

As you bend forward, your objective is not only to maintain your balance, but also to maintain your bent knee pointing outwards. This targets the flexibility of the hip sockets, especially the one of the non-weight-bearing leg.

celebrity couples

Season 1

- Trista Rehn Sutter – Partner: Louis van Amstel
- Evander Holyfield – Partner: Edyta Sliwinska
- Rachel Hunter – Partner: Jonathan Roberts
- Joey McIntyre – Partner: Ashly DelGrosso
- John O'Hurley – Partner: Charlotte Jorgensen
- Kelly Monaco – Partner: Alec Mazo (WINNERS)

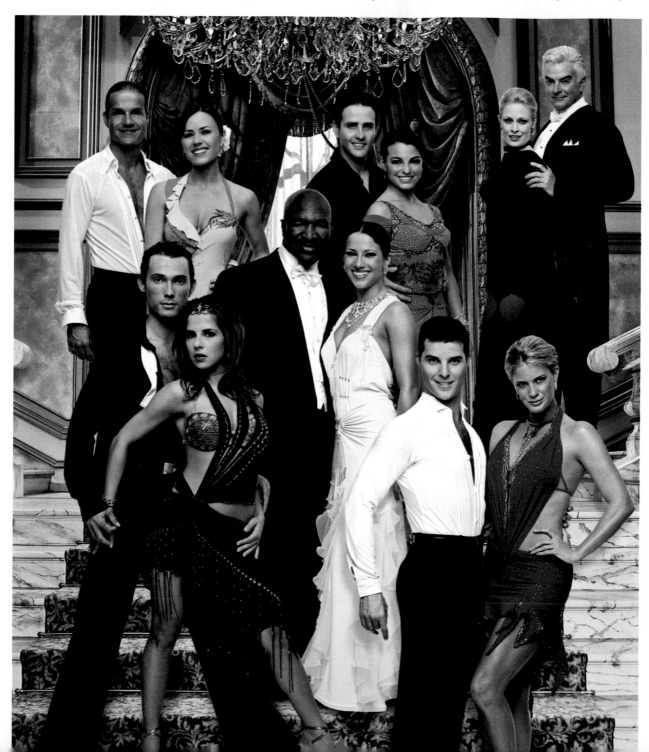

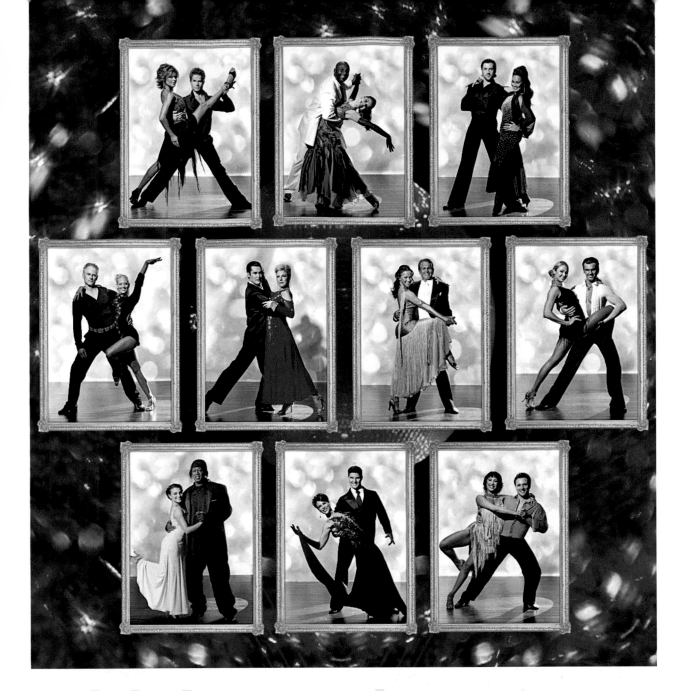

celebrity couples

Season 2

- Kenny Mayne – Partner: Andrea Hale
- Tatum O'Neal – Partner: Nick Kosovich
- Giselle Fernandez – Partner: Jonathan Roberts
- Master P – Partner: Ashly DelGrosso
- Tia Carrere – Partner: Maksim Chmerkovskiy

- George Hamilton – Partner: Edyta Sliwinska
- Lisa Rinna – Partner: Louis van Amstel
- Stacy Keibler – Partner: Tony Dovolani
- Jerry Rice – Partner: Anna Trebunskaya
- Drew Lachey – Partner: Cheryl Burke (WINNERS)

celebrity couples

Season 3

- Tucker Carlson – Partner: Elena Grinenko
- Shanna Moakler – Partner: Jesse DeSoto
- Harry Hamlin – Partner: Ashly DelGrosso
- Vivica A. Fox – Partner: Nick Kosovich
- Willa Ford – Partner: Maksim Chmerkovskiy
- Sara Evans – Partner: Tony Dovolani

- Jerry Springer – Partner: Kym Johnson
- Monique Coleman – Partner: Louis van Amstel
- Joey Lawrence – Partner: Edyta Sliwinska
- Mario Lopez – Partner: Karina Smirnoff
- Emmitt Smith – Partner: Cheryl Burke (WINNERS)

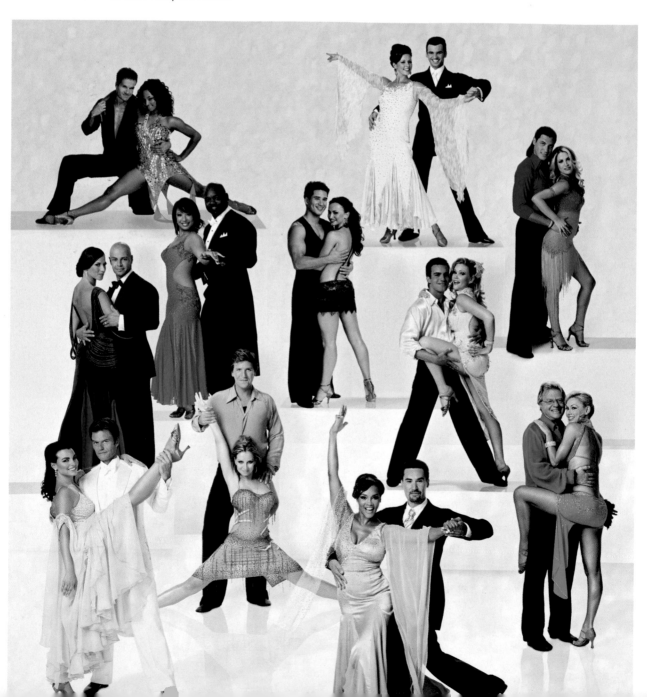

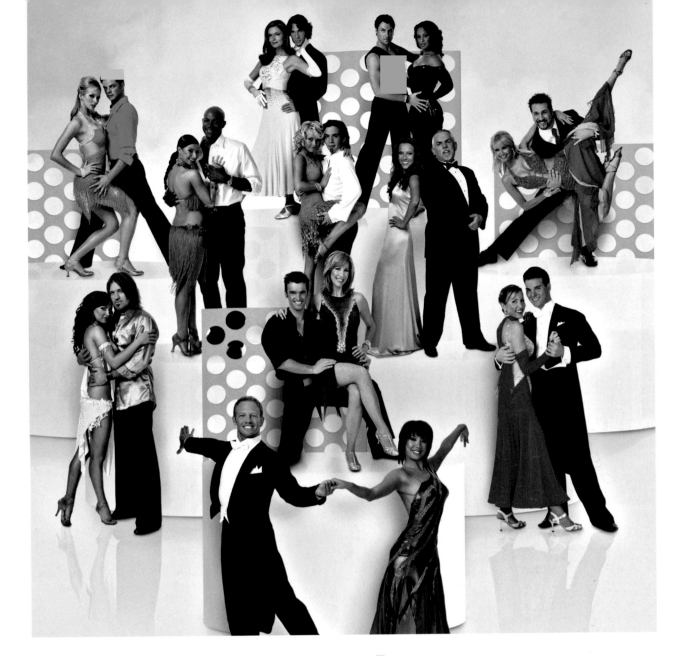

celebrity couples

Season 4

- Paulina Porizkova – Partner: Alec Mazo
- Shandi Finnessey – Partner: Brian Fortuna
- Leeza Gibbons – Partner: Tony Dovolani
- Clyde Drexler – Partner: Elena Grinenko
- Heather Mills – Partner: Jonathan Roberts
- John Ratzenberger – Partner: Edyta Sliwinska
- Billy Ray Cyrus – Partner: Karina Smirnoff
- Ian Ziering – Partner: Cheryl Burke
- Laila Ali – Partner: Maksim Chmerkovskiy
- Joey Fatone – Partner: Kym Johnson
- Apolo Anton Ohno – Partner: Julianne Hough (WINNERS)

show results

SEASON/SHOW/ DANCE NO	COUPLE	DANCE	SONG	ARTIST	JUDGE'S SCORES			
Season 1								
Show 1, dance 1	Joey and Ashly	Cha-cha	*Crazy in Love*	Beyoncé	7	7	6	20
Show 1, dance 2	Rachel and Jonathan	Waltz	*Three Times a Lady*	The Commodores	7	6	7	20
Show 1, dance 3	John and Charlotte	Cha-cha	*September*	Earth, Wind and Fire	7	7	6	20
Show 1, dance 4	Evander and Edyta	Cha-cha	*Respect*	Aretha Franklin	5	7	6	18
Show 1, dance 5	Trista and Louis	Waltz	*Come Away With Me*	Norah Jones	6	6	6	18
Show 1, dance 6	Kelly and Alec	Waltz	*I Have Nothing*	Whitney Houston	5	4	4	13
Show 2, dance 1	Rachel and Jonathan	Rumba	*Don't Want To Miss A Thing*	Aerosmith	8	8	8	24
Show 2, dance 2	Joey and Ashly	Quickstep	*You're The One That I Want*	John Travolta and Olivia Newton John	8	7	6	21
Show 2, dance 3	Trista and Louis	Rumba	*Endless Love*	Lionel Richie	6	7	6	19
Show 2, dance 4	John and Charlotte	Quickstep	*Let's Face The Music and Dance*	Frank Sinatra	8	9	9	26
Show 2, dance 5	Kelly and Alec	Rumba	*Hero*	Enrique Iglesias	5	6	6	17
Show 2, dance 6	Evander and Edyta	Quickstep	*It Don't Mean A Thing If It Ain't Got That Swing*	Ross Mitchell	5	4	5	14
Show 3, dance 1	Evander and Edyta	Jive	*Reet Petite*	Jackie Wilson	5	4	4	13
Show 3, dance 2	Rachel and Jonathan	Tango	*Toxic*	Britney Spears	8	8	9	25
Show 3, dance 3	Kelly and Alec	Jive	*Footloose*	Kenny Loggins	6	7	8	21
Show 3, dance 4	John and Charlotte	Tango	*Dance With Me*	Deborah Morgan	9	8	7	24
Show 3, dance 5	Joey and Ashly	Jive	*I'm Still Standing*	Elton John	7	7	8	22
Show 4, dance 1	Joey and Ashly	Samba	*Tequila*	Strictly Ballroom	7	6	7	20
Show 4, dance 2	Rachel and Jonathan	Samba	*Soul Bassa Nova*	Quincy Jones and Orchestra	7	9	9	25
Show 4, dance 3	John and Charlotte	Samba	*Just the Two of Us*	Grover Washington Jr.	7	8	6	21
Show 4, dance 4	Kelly and Alec	Samba	*Bailamos*	Enrique Iglesias	9	9	8	26
Show 4, dance 5	All Couples	Viennese Waltz	*I Got You Babe*	Sonny and Cher				NONE
Show 5, dance 1	John and Charlotte	Paso Doble	*Spanish Gypsy Dance (aka Espana Cani)*	Erich Kunzel	9	9	9	27
Show 5, dance 2	Kelly and Alec	Paso Doble	*Bamboleo*	Gypsy Kings	8	7	7	22
Show 5, dance 3	Joey and Ashly	Paso Doble	*Eye of The Tiger*	Survivor	8	6	6	20
Show 5, dance 4	John and Charlotte	Foxtrot	*Let There Be Love*	Nat King Cole	9	9	9	27
Show 5, dance 5	Kelly and Alec	Foxtrot	*Don't Know Why*	Norah Jones	9	8	8	25
Show 5, dance 6	Joey and Ashly	Foxtrot	*Big Spender*	Shirley Bassey	6	8	8	22
Show 6, dance 1	John and Charlotte	Quickstep	*Let's Face The Music and Dance*	Frank Sinatra	9	9	9	27
Show 6, dance 2	Kelly and Alec	Samba	*Bailamos*	Enrique Iglesias	7	9	9	25
Show 6, dance 3	John and Charlotte	Freestyle	*I'm So Excited*	Pointer Sisters	9	9	9	27
Show 6, dance 4	Kelly and Alec	Freestyle	*Let's Get Loud*	Jennifer Lopez	10	10	10	30
Show 6, dance 5	Trista and Louis,	Group Dances	*Endless Love*	Lionel Richie				NONE
Show 6, dance 6	Evander and Edyta	Group Dances	*Reet Petite*	Jackie Wilson				NONE
Show 6, dance 7	Rachel and Jonathan	Group Dances	*Toxic*	Britney Spears				NONE
Show 6, dance 8	Joey and Ashly	Group Dances	*Crazy in Love*	Beyoncé				NONE
Special:								
Dance 1	Kelly and Alec	Cha-cha	*Lady Marmalade*	Christina Aguilera, Pink, Mya, Little Kim				
Dance 2	John and Charlotte	Waltz	*You Light Up My Life*	Whitney Houston				
Dance 3	Charlotte and Nick	Waltz	*Ain't No Sunshine When She's Gone*	Bill Withers				
Dance 4	Kelly and Alec	Quickstep	*Diamond's Are A Girl's Best Friend*	Marilyn Monroe				
Dance 5	John and Charlotte	Rumba	*The Look of Love*	Dusty Springfield				
Dance 6	Louis and Ashly	Jive	*Proud Mary*	Tina Turner				
Dance 7	Jonathan and Anna	Foxtrot	*Fields of Gold*	Sting				
Dance 8	Alec and Edyta	Samba	*Ain't It Funny*	Jennifer Lopez				
Dance 9	Kelly and John	Group Dances	*Don't Stop Me Now*	Queen				
Dance 10	Kelly and Alec	Freestyle	*Get the Party Started*	Pink				
Dance 11	John and Charlotte	Freestyle	*I Am What I Am*	Gloria Gaynor				
Season 2								
Show 1, dance 1	Drew and Cheryl	Cha-cha	*She Bangs*	Ricky Martin	8	8	8	24
Show 1, dance 2	Giselle and Jonathan	Waltz	*I Never Loved a Man*	Aretha Franklin	7	8	8	23
Show 1, dance 3	Tatum and Nick	Waltz	*What The World Needs Now*	Jackie DeShannon	8	7	8	23
Show 1, dance 4	Stacy and Tony	Waltz	*I Wonder Why*	Curtis Stigers	8	6	8	22
Show 1, dance 5	Jerry and Anna	Cha-cha	*I Like It Like That*	Blackout Allstars	7	7	7	21
Show 1, dance 6	Tia and Maks	Waltz	*What A Wonderful World*	Ross Mitchell	6	7	7	20
Show 1, dance 7	Lisa and Louis	Waltz	*Natural Woman*	Carole King	5	7	7	19
Show 1, dance 8	George and Edyta	Cha-cha	*Oye Como Va*	Santana	7	5	6	18
Show 1, dance 9	Kenny and Andrea	Cha-cha	*Hot Stuff*	Donna Summer	4	5	4	13
Show 1, dance 10	P and Ashly	Cha-cha	*I Want You Back*	Jackson 5	4	4	4	12
Show 1, dance 11	Pro Rumba and Quickstep Dancers	Artists/Dancers	*The Look of Love*	Burt Bacharach				NONE

SEASON/SHOW/ DANCE NO	COUPLE	DANCE	SONG	ARTIST	Carrie Ann Inaba	Len Goodman	Bruno Tonioli	Total
					JUDGE'S SCORES			
Show 1, dance 12	Pro Rumba and Quickstep Dancers	Artists/Dancers	*Sign Your Name, Mack the Knife*	Terence Trent D'Arby, Frank Sinatra	NONE			
Show 2, dance 1	Stacy and Tony	Rumba	*I'm Like a Bird*	Nelly Furtado	9	10	10	29
Show 2, dance 2	Drew and Cheryl	Quickstep	*Neutron Dance*	Pointer Sisters	9	9	9	27
Show 2, dance 3	Giselle and Jonathan	Rumba	*Take My Breath Away*	Berlin	8	8	8	24
Show 2, dance 4	Jerry and Anna	Quickstep	*If My Friends Could See Me Now*	Sammy Davis Jr.	7	8	8	23
Show 2, dance 5	Tia and Maks	Rumba	*Emotion*	Destiny's Child	7	8	7	22
Show 2, dance 6	George and Edyta	Quickstep	*Top Hat, White Tie, and Tails*	Fred Astaire	8	7	7	22
Show 2, dance 7	Lisa and Louis	Rumba	*Your Song*	Elton John	6	7	7	20
Show 2, dance 8	Tatum and Nick	Rumba	*Careless Whisper*	George Michael	5	6	6	17
Show 2, dance 9	P and Ashly	Quickstep	*Zoot Suit Riot*	Cherry Poppin' Daddies	6	5	5	16
Show 2, dance 10	Pro Couples	Artists/Dancers	*Get Your Shine On*	Jesse McCartney	NONE			
Show 2, dance 11	Pro Lindyhop (Ryan and Jenny)	Artists/Dancers	*That Ole Black Magic*	Sammy Davis Jr.	NONE			
Show 3, dance 1	Drew and Cheryl	Jive	*Crazy Little Thing Called Love*	Queen	9	9	9	27
Show 3, dance 2	Stacy and Tony	Tango	*Cell Block Tango*	Chicago Soundtrack	9	9	9	27
Show 3, dance 3	Tia and Maks	Tango	*Por Una Cabeza*	The Tango Project	9	8	9	26
Show 3, dance 4	Lisa and Louis	Jive	*Jailhouse Rock*	Elvis Presley	8	9	8	25
Show 3, dance 5	Giselle and Jonathan	Tango	*Hernando's Hideaway*	Victor Silvester	7	8	7	22
Show 3, dance 6	George and Edyta	Tango	*La Cumparsita*	Danny Malando	7	7	8	22
Show 3, dance 7	Jerry and Anna	Jive	*Do You Love Me*	The Contours	7	6	6	19
Show 3, dance 8	P and Ashly	Jive	*Saturday Night's Alright For Fighting*	Elton John	6	4	4	14
Show 3, dance 9	Pro Paso Doble	Artists/Dancers (Anna, Jonathan, Cheryl, Edyta, Louis, Tony, Ashly, Maks)	*Gonna Fly Now*	Bill Conti	NONE			
Show 3, dance 10	Breakdance Act	Artists/Dancers	*Hey Mama*	Black Eyed Peas	NONE			
Show 4, dance 1	Drew and Cheryl	Paso Doble	*Thriller*	Michael Jackson	9	9	10	28
Show 4, dance 2	Stacy and Tony	Foxtrot	*Cold Cold Heart*	Norah Jones	8	9	9	26
Show 4, dance 3	Lisa and Louis	Paso Doble	*The Final Countdown*	Europe	9	9	8	26
Show 4, dance 4	Tia and Maks	Foxtrot	*Dream A Little Dream*	Mama Cass	9	8	8	25
Show 4, dance 5	Jerry and Anna	Paso Doble	*Espana Cani*	Erich Kunzel	8	8	8	24
Show 4, dance 6	George and Edyta	Paso Doble	*Matador Paso*	Andy Fortuna	7	7	7	21
Show 4, dance 7	P and Ashly	Paso Doble	*Don't Let Me Be Misunderstood*	The Animals	4	2	2	8
Show 4, dance 8	Pro Salsa Dancers	Artists/Dancers	*Cha Cha*	Chelo	NONE			
Show 4, dance 9	Pro Dancers	Artists/Dancers	*Don't Cha*	Pussy Cat Dolls	NONE			
Show 4, dance 10	Jonathan and Anna	Artists/Dancers	*Sway*	Pussy Cat Dolls	NONE			
Show 4, dance 11	Pro Mambo Dancers	Artists/Dancers	*Rank*	Tito Puente	NONE			
Show 5, dance 1	Stacy and Tony	Samba	*Bootylicious*	Destiny's Child	10	10	10	30
Show 5, dance 2	Drew and Cheryl	Samba	*Dirrty*	Christina Aguilera	9	9	9	27
Show 5, dance 3	Lisa and Louis	Samba	*Le Freak*	Chic	7	9	9	25
Show 5, dance 4	George and Edyta	Samba	*Conga*	Gloria Estefan	8	8	8	24
Show 5, dance 5	Jerry and Anna	Samba	*For Once In My Life*	Stevie Wonder	7	8	8	23
Show 5, dance 6	Tia and Maks	Samba	*No More Tears (Enough is Enough)*	Donna Summer	7	7	8	22
Show 5, dance 7	Louis and Cheryl	Artists/Dancers	*Copacabana*	Barry Manilow	NONE			
Show 5, dance 8	Pro Dancers	Artists/Dancers	*Unchained Melody*	Barry Manilow	NONE			
Show 5, dance 9	All Couples	Group Dances	*Rythm Is Going To Get You*	Gloria Estefan	NONE			
Show 6, dance 1	Drew and Cheryl	Tango	*Shut Up*	Black Eyed Peas	10	10	10	30
Show 6, dance 2	Stacy and Tony	Jive	*Wake Me Up Before You Go Go*	Wham!	10	10	10	30
Show 6, dance 3	Lisa and Louis	Quickstep	*9 to 5*	Chic	9	9	9	27
Show 6, dance 4	Jerry and Anna	Paso Doble	*Espana Cani*	Erich Kunzel	8	7	8	23
Show 6, dance 5	George and Edyta	Rumba	*Perhaps Perhaps Perhaps*	Doris Day	8	7	8	23
Show 6, dance 6	Pro Dancers	Group Dances	*Faith, La Cumparsita, My Heart*	Various	NONE			
Show 6, dance 7	Pro Dancers (Maks' Students)	Artists/Dancers	*Mambo #5*	Lou Bega	NONE			
Show 6, dance 8	Pro Dancers	Artists/Dancers	*Unwritten*	Natasha Bedingfield	NONE			
Show 6, dance 9	Tony and Cheryl	Artists/Dancers	*I've Had the Time of My Life*	Bill Medley	NONE			
Show 6, dance 10	All Couples	Group Dances	*Fallin'*	Alicia Keys	NONE			
Show 7, dance 1	Stacy and Tony	Quickstep	*You Can't Hurry Love*	Phil Collins	9	9	9	27
Show 7, dance 2	Lisa and Louis	Foxtrot	*Fever*	Peggy Lee	8	9	9	26
Show 7, dance 3	Drew and Cheryl	Foxtrot	*It Had To Be You*	Harry Connick Jr.	9	9	8	26
Show 7, dance 4	Jerry and Anna	Tango	*One Way Or Another*	Blondie	7	7	6	20
Show 7, dance 5	Drew and Cheryl	Rumba	*Total Eclipse Of The Heart*	Bonnie Tyler	10	9	10	29
Show 7, dance 6	Stacy and Tony	Cha-cha	*Since U Been Gone*	Kelly Clarkson	9	10	9	28
Show 7, dance 7	Lisa and Louis	Cha-cha	*Material Girl*	Madonna	9	9	9	27
Show 7, dance 8	Jerry and Anna	Rumba	*Unbreak My Heart*	Toni Braxton	7	7	7	21
Show 7, dance 9	Alec and Edyta	Artists/Dancers	*Save the Last Dance*	Michael Buble	NONE			
Show 7, dance 10	Nick and Andrea	Artists/Dancers	*Moondance*	Michael Buble	NONE			

SEASON/SHOW/ DANCE NO	COUPLE	DANCE	SONG	ARTIST	Carrie Ann Inaba	Len Goodman	Bruno Tonioli	Total
								JUDGE'S SCORES
Show 7, dance 11	Tom Bergeron and Ashly	Group Dances	Get Happy	Judy Garland				NONE
Show 8, dance 1	Jerry and Anna	Foxtrot	Why Don't You Do Right	Julie London	9	9	8	26
Show 8, dance 2	Stacy and Tony	Jive	Wake Me Up Before You Go Go	Wham!	10	10	10	30
Show 8, dance 3	Drew and Cheryl	Paso Doble	Thriller	Michael Jackson	10	10	10	30
Show 8, dance 4	Jerry and Anna	Freestyle	Celebration	Kool And The Gang	9	9	9	27
Show 8, dance 5	Stacy and Tony	Freestyle	Staying Alive	Bee Gees	8	8	9	25
Show 8, dance 6	Drew and Cheryl	Freestyle	Save a Horse, Ride A Cowboy	Big and Rich	10	10	10	30
Show 8, dance 7	Jerry and Anna	Cha-cha	Think	Aretha Franklin	9	9	9	27
Show 8, dance 8	Stacy and Tony	Samba	Livin La Vida Loca	Ricky Martin	10	10	10	30
Show 8, dance 9	Drew and Cheryl	Jive	Hound Dog	Elvis Presley	9	9	9	27
Show 8, dance 10	Kenny, Tatum, Giselle, P	Group Dances	Hot Stuff, What the World Needs Now, Take My Breath Away	Various				NONE
Show 8, dance 11	Tia, George, Lisa	Group Dances	Por Una Cabeza, Top Hat White Tie, Jailhouse Rock	Various				NONE
Show 8, dance 12	All Couples	Group Dances	I Wanna Dance With Somebody	Whitney Houston				NONE
Show 8, dance 13	Samantha Harris and Jonathan	Group Dances	Delirious	Prince				NONE
Show 8, dance 14	Pro Couples	Artists/Dancers	Be Without You	Mary J. Blige				NONE
Show 8, dance 15	Salsa dancers	Artists/Dancers	Family Affair	Mary J. Blige				NONE
Season 3								
Show 1, dance 1	Mario and Karina	Cha-cha	Walkin' on the Sun	Smash Mouth	9	8	9	27
Show 1, dance 2	Emmitt and Cheryl	Cha-cha	Son of A Preacher Man	Dusty Springfield	8	8	8	24
Show 1, dance 3	Willa and Maks	Foxtrot	TRUE	Spandau Ballet	7	7	8	22
Show 1, dance 4	Vivica and Nick	Foxtrot	I Just Wanna Make Love to You	Etta James	6	8	8	22
Show 1, dance 5	Joey and Edyta	Cha-cha	I like the Way You Move	Body Rockers	7	7	7	21
Show 1, dance 6	Monique and Louis	Foxtrot	Baby Love	Diana Ross	6	6	7	19
Show 1, dance 7	Shanna and Jesse	Foxtrot	Saving All My Love	Whitney Houston	7	5	6	18
Show 1, dance 8	Harry and Ashly	Cha-cha	Disco Inferno	The Trammps	5	6	6	17
Show 1, dance 9	Jerry and Kym	Cha-cha	Hey Daddy	Della Reese	5	5	6	16
Show 1, dance 10	Sara and Tony	Foxtrot	Mandy	Barry Manilow	5	5	5	15
Show 1, dance 11	Tucker and Elena	Cha-cha	Dancing in the Street	David Bowie/Mick Jagger	5	4	3	12
Show 1, dance 12	Pro Couples	Artists/Dancers	She's A Lady	Tom Jones				NONE
Show 1, dance 13	Louis and Karina	Artists/Dancers	It's Not Unusual	Tom Jones				NONE
Show 1, dance 14	Pro Dancers	Group Dances	Misirlou	Dick Dale and his Del Tones				NONE
Show 2, dance 1	Joey and Edyta	Quickstep	I Got Rythm	Ella Fitzgerald	10	9	10	29
Show 2, dance 2	Monique and Louis	Mambo	Bop To The Top	High School Musical	9	8	9	26
Show 2, dance 3	Vivica and Nick	Mambo	Betece	Africando All Stars	8	8	8	24
Show 2, dance 4	Emmitt and Cheryl	Quickstep	Black Horse and The Cherry Tree	KT Tunstall	8	8	8	24
Show 2, dance 5	Willa and Maks	Mambo	Get Busy	Sean Paul	7	8	8	23
Show 2, dance 6	Shanna and Jesse	Mambo	Jump	Kriss Kross	8	7	7	22
Show 2, dance 7	Harry and Ashly	Quickstep	Lust For Life	Iggy Pop	7	7	7	21
Show 2, dance 8	Mario and Karina	Quickstep	Do Your Thing	Basement Jaxx	7	6	8	21
Show 2, dance 9	Sara and Tony	Mambo	Papa Loves Mambo	Perry Como	7	7	7	21
Show 2, dance 10	Jerry and Kym	Quickstep	Sing Sing Sing	The Andrews Sisters	7	6	6	19
Show 2, dance 11	Maks and Cheryl	Artists/Dancers	I Wanna Know What Love Is	Julio Iglesias				NONE
Show 2, dance 12	Jordi Caballero and Claudia Velsco Tango	Artists/Dancers	Dance Away	Roxy Music				NONE
Show 2, dance 13	Pro Dancers	Group Dances	Rebel Yell	Billy Idol				NONE
Show 3, dance 1	Vivica and Nick	Tango	Hey Sexy Lady	Shaggy	9	9	9	27
Show 3, dance 2	Monique and Louis	Jive	The Heat is On	Glen Frey	9	9	9	27
Show 3, dance 3	Sara and Tony	Jive	These Boots Are Made For Walking	Nancy Sinatra	8	9	8	25
Show 3, dance 4	Harry and Ashly	Tango	Santa Maria	Gotan Project	7	8	7	22
Show 3, dance 5	Willa and Maks	Jive	SOS	Rihanna	7	7	8	22
Show 3, dance 6	Mario and Karina	Tango	What You Waiting For	Gwen Stefani	8	6	8	22
Show 3, dance 7	Joey and Edyta	Jive	Blue Suede Shoes	Elvis Presley	8	6	8	22
Show 3, dance 8	Jerry and Kym	Tango	Hernando's Hideaway	Ella Fitzgerald	7	7	7	21
Show 3, dance 9	Emmitt and Cheryl	Tango	Simply Irresistible	Robert Palmer	7	6	6	19
Show 3, dance 10	Pro Dancers	Artists/Dancers	I Don't Feel Like Dancin	Scissor Sisters				NONE
Show 3, dance 11	Jesse and Cheryl	Artists/Dancers	Take Your Mama	Scissor Sisters				NONE
Show 4, dance 1	Mario and Karina	Paso Doble	Cancion Del Mariachi	Desperado Los Lobos & A Banderas	10	9	10	29
Show 4, dance 2	Willa and Maks	Waltz	You Light Up My Life	Leann Rimes	9	9	10	28
Show 4, dance 3	Joey and Edyta	Waltz	Take It To The Limit	The Eagles	9	9	9	27

SEASON/SHOW/ DANCE NO	COUPLE	DANCE	SONG	ARTIST	Carrie Ann Inaba	Len Goodman	Bruno Tonioli	Total
					JUDGE'S SCORES			
Show 4, dance 4	Vivica and Nick	Paso Doble	It's My Life	Bon Jovi	8	8	8	24
Show 4, dance 5	Emmitt and Cheryl	Paso Doble	Espani Cani	Erich Kunzel	8	8	8	24
Show 4, dance 6	Monique and Louis	Waltz	If I Were Painting	Kenny Rogers	8	8	8	24
Show 4, dance 7	Jerry and Kym	Waltz	Tennessee Waltz	Patti Page	7	7	8	22
Show 4, dance 8	Sara and Tony	Paso Doble	Phantom Of The Opera	Phantom Soundtrack	6	7	7	20
Show 4, dance 9	Tony and Elena	Artists/Dancers	Can't Hate You Anymore	Nick Lachey				NONE
Show 4, dance 10	Back up dancers	Artists/Dancers	My Way	Los Lonely Boys				NONE
Show 4, dance 11	Delgrosso Sisters	Artists/Dancers	Heatwave	Martha Reeves and the Vandellas				NONE
Show 5, dance 1	Willa and Maks	Rumba	Every Breath You Take	Police	9	9	9	27
Show 5, dance 2	Emmitt and Cheryl	Samba	Cha Cha	Chelo	9	9	9	27
Show 5, dance 3	Mario and Karina	Rumba	The Way You Look Tonight	Michael Buble	9	9	9	27
Show 5, dance 4	Monique and Louis	Rumba	So Nice	Bebel Gilberto	9	9	9	27
Show 5, dance 5	Joey and Edyta	Samba	Freedom	George Michael	8	8	9	25
Show 5, dance 6	Sara and Tony	Samba	I Wish	Stevie Wonder	8	8	8	24
Show 5, dance 7	Jerry and Kym	Samba	Eso Beso	Paul Anka	8	8	8	24
Show 5, dance 8	Kym and Edyta	Artists/Dancers	Hot Legs	Rod Stewart				NONE
Show 5, dance 9	Kym and Edyta	Artists/Dancers	Fooled Around and Fell in Love	Rod Stewart				NONE
Show 5, dance 10	Pro Disco Dancers	Artists/Dancers	Boogie Wonderland	Earth Wind and Fire				NONE
Show 6, dance 1	Mario and Karina	Mambo	Ran Kan Kan	Tito Puente	9	9	10	28
Show 6, dance 2	Emmitt and Cheryl	Jive	Lewis Boogie Blues	Walk The Line Soundtrack	8	8	9	25
Show 6, dance 3	Joey and Edyta	Rumba	Father Figure	George Michael	8	8	8	24
Show 6, dance 4	Monique and Louis	Samba	ABC	Jackson 5	9	7	7	23
Show 6, dance 5	Jerry and Kym	Paso Doble	Habanera	Charlotte Church	7	6	5	18
Show 6, dance 6	Maks, Karina, Tony, Elena	Artists/Dancers	All Night Long	Lionel Richie				NONE
Show 6, dance 7	Maks, Karina, Tony, Elena	Artists/Dancers	I Call it Love	Lionel Richie				NONE
Show 6, dance 8	Nick and Lena Kosovich	Artists/Dancers	The Show Must Go On	Queen				NONE
Show 6, dance 9	All Couples	Group Dancers	Don't Stop Til You Get Enough	Michael Jackson				NONE
Show 6, dance 10	Pro Dancers	Group Dancers	Rock Around the Clock, Right Now, Espana Cani, Tired of Being Alone	Various				NONE
Show 7, dance 1	Mario and Karina	Foxtrot	I Just Wanna Be Loved By You	Marilyn Monroe	10	9	10	29
Show 7, dance 2	Joey and Edyta	Foxtrot	Singing in the Rain	Gene Kelly	10	9	10	29
Show 7, dance 3	Emmitt and Cheryl	Waltz	Hushabye Mountain	Bobbie Gentry	10	9	9	28
Show 7, dance 4	Monique and Louis	Quickstep	Luck Be a Lady	Frank Sinatra	9	9	9	27
Show 7, dance 5	Jerry and Kym	Foxtrot	My Way	Frank Sinatra	8	8	8	24
Show 7, dance 6	Emmitt and Cheryl	Mambo	Que Bueno Baila Usted	Oscar D'Leon	10	10	9	29
Show 7, dance 7	Joey and Edyta	Mambo	Mambo Number 5	Lou Bega	9	9	10	28
Show 7, dance 8	Monique and Louis	Paso Doble	The Reflex	Duran Duran	9	9	9	27
Show 7, dance 9	Mario and Karina	Jive	Shake A Tailfeather	Ray Charles Blues Brothers	9	9	9	27
Show 7, dance 10	Jerry and Kym	Mambo	Annie I'm Not Your Daddy	Kid Creole and the Coconuts	7	8	7	22
Show 7, dance 11	Alec and Edyta	Artists/Dancers	Rose Garden	Martina McBride				NONE
Show 7, dance 12	Back-up dancers	Artists/Dancers	This One's For The Girl	Martina McBride				NONE
Show 7, dance 13	Maks' students	Artists/Dancers	Billie Jean	Michael Jackson				NONE
Show 8, dance 1	Joey and Edyta	Tango	The Addams Family	TV Theme	10	9	9	28
Show 8, dance 2	Mario and Karina	Waltz	Dark Waltz	Hayley Westenra	9	9	10	28
Show 8, dance 3	Emmitt and Cheryl	Foxtrot	Witchcraft	Frank Sinatra	8	8	9	25
Show 8, dance 4	Monique and Louis	Tango	Somebody's Watching Me	Royal Gigolos	8	8	8	24
Show 8, dance 5	Mario and Karina	Samba	Superstition	Stevie Wonder	10	9	10	29
Show 8, dance 6	Monique and Louis	Cha-cha	Ghostbusters	Ray Parker Jr.	9	10	10	29
Show 8, dance 7	Emmitt and Cheryl	Rumba	Spooky	Dusty Springfield	9	10	10	29
Show 8, dance 8	Joey and Edyta	Paso Doble	Sympathy For The Devil	Rolling Stones	9	8	9	26
Show 8, dance 9	Victor and Anna	Artists/Dancers	Without You	Il Divo				NONE
Show 8, dance 10	Pro Dancers	Artists/Dancers	Fame	Performed by Willa Ford				NONE
Show 8, dance 11	SWOP Dancers	Artists/Dancers	Crazy In Love	Beyoncé				NONE
Show 8, dance 12	Back up dancers	Artists/Dancers	West End Girls	Pet Shop Boys				NONE
Show 9, dance 1	Mario and Karina	Tango	Whatever Lola Wants	Sarah Vaughan	10	10	10	30
Show 9, dance 2	Emmitt and Cheryl	Waltz	At This Moment	Billy Vera and The Beaters	9	10	10	29
Show 9, dance 3	Joey and Edyta	Quickstep	42nd Street	Lee Roy Reams	9	10	10	29
Show 9, dance 4	Emmitt and Cheryl	Cha-cha	Dance To The Music	Sly and The Family Stone	10	10	10	30
Show 9, dance 5	Joey and Edyta	Rumba	Eternal Flame	Bangles	10	10	10	30
Show 9, dance 6	Mario and Karina	Cha-cha	Bad	Michael Jackson	10	9	10	29
Show 9, dance 7	Jonathan, Anna, Maks, Kym, Tony, Elena	Artists/Dancers	James Bond Theme	John Barry				NONE
Show 9, dance 8	Group Tour dance, Willa, Maks, Harry, Ashly, Lisa, Louis, Joey M, Kym	Artists/Dancers	Footloose	Kenny Loggins				NONE
Show 10, dance 1	Emmitt and Cheryl	Samba	Sir Duke	Stevie Wonder	10	10	10	30
Show 10, dance 2	Mario and Karina	Samba	Sir Duke	Stevie Wonder	10	9	10	29
Show 10, dance 3	Emmitt and Cheryl	Mambo	Que Bueno Baila Usted	Oscar D'Leon	10	10	10	30

show results 243

show results

SEASON/SHOW/ DANCE NO	COUPLE	DANCE	SONG	ARTIST	Carrie Ann Inaba	Len Goodman	Bruno Tonioli	Total
					JUDGE'S SCORES			
Show 10, dance 4	Mario and Karina	Paso Doble	*Cancion Del Mariachi*	Desperado Los Lobos & A Banderas	10	10	10	30
Show 10, dance 5	Emmitt and Cheryl	Freestyle	*You Can't Touch This*	MC Hammer	10	10	10	30
Show 10, dance 6	Mario and Karina	Freestyle	*It Takes Two*	Rob Base and DJ EZ Rock	10	10	9	29
Show 10, dance 7	Tucker, Shanna, Harry and Vivica	Group Dancers	*Dancing in the Street, Jump, Lust for Life, It's My Life*	Various				NONE
Show 10, dance 8	Willa, Sara, Jerry, Monique, Joey	Group Dancers	*Every Breath You Take, These Boots Were Made For Walking, Esto Beso, Heat Is On, Singing in the Rain*	Various				NONE
Season 4								
Show 1, dance 1	Joey and Kym	Cha-cha	*You Should Be Dancing*	Bee Gees	8	8	8	24
Show 1, dance 2	Laila and Maks	Foxtrot	*How Sweet It Is*	Marvin Gaye	7	8	8	23
Show 1, dance 3	Ian and Cheryl	Cha-cha	*Mony Mony*	Billy Idol	7	7	7	21
Show 1, dance 4	Apolo and Julianne	Cha-cha	*Let's Hear It For The Boy*	Deniece Williams	7	7	7	21
Show 1, dance 5	Paulina and Alec	Foxtrot	*Too Darn Hot*	Ella Fitzgerald	6	6	7	19
Show 1, dance 6	Shandi and Brian	Foxtrot	*The Power of Love*	Huey Lewis and The News	6	6	7	19
Show 1, dance 7	Heather and Jonathan	Foxtrot	*Cheek to Cheek*	Ella Fitzgerald	6	6	6	18
Show 1, dance 8	John and Edyta	Cha-cha	*Chain of Fools*	Aretha Franklin	6	5	6	17
Show 1, dance 9	Clyde and Elena	Cha-cha	*I Was Made to Love Her*	Stevie Wonder	6	5	5	16
Show 1, dance 10	Leeza and Tony	Foxtrot	*Strangers In The Night*	Frank Sinatra	5	5	5	15
Show 1, dance 11	Billy Ray and Karina	Cha-cha	*I Want My Mullet Back*	Billy Ray Cyrus	5	4	4	13
Show 1, dance 13	Pro Dancers - Cha Cha	Cha-cha	*Ballroom Blitz*	Tia Carrere				NONE
Show 2, dance 1	Laila and Maks	Mambo	*Maracaibo Oriental*	Benny More	9	9	9	27
Show 2, dance 2	Apolo and Julianne	Quickstep	*Two Hearts*	Phil Collins	8	9	9	26
Show 2, dance 3	Heather and Jonathan	Mambo	*Hey Mambo*	Dean Martin	8	8	8	24
Show 2, dance 4	Joey and Kym	Quickstep	*Tell Her About It*	Billy Joel	8	8	8	24
Show 2, dance 5	Ian and Cheryl	Quickstep	*Don't Get Me Wrong*	The Pretenders	7	8	7	22
Show 2, dance 6	Leeza and Tony	Mambo	*Independent Women*	Destiny's Child	7	7	7	21
Show 2, dance 7	Paulina and Alec	Mambo	*La Bamba*	Los Lobos	7	7	7	21
Show 2, dance 8	Billy Ray and Karina	Quickstep	*Ring of Fire*	Johnny Cash	7	7	7	21
Show 2, dance 9	John and Edyta	Quickstep	*The Lady Is A Tramp*	Sammy Davis Jr.	7	7	7	21
Shwo 2, dance 10	Shandi and Brian	Mambo	*Right Now*	Pussycat Dolls	6	7	7	20
Show 2, dance 11	Clyde and Elena	Quickstep	*Higher and Higher*	Jackie Wilson	6	6	6	18
Show 2, dance 12	Pro Dancers	Jive	*Don't Stop Me Now*	Queen				NONE
Show 2, dance 13	Jonathan, Cheryl, Anna, and Pavlo Barsuk	Artists/Dancers	*I Say A Little Prayer For You*	Dionne Warwick				NONE
Show 2, dance 14	Back up dancers, Claudia Velasco and Yesenia Adame	Artists/Dancers	*Do You Know The Way To San Jose*	Dionne Warwick				NONE
Show 3, dance 1	Joey and Kym	Tango	*Star Wars Cantina Band*	Meco	8	8	8	24
Show 3, dance 2	Ian and Cheryl	Jive	*Hard Headed Woman*	Elvis Presley	8	8	8	24
Show 3, dance 3	Leeza and Tony	Tango	*Jealousy*	Billy Fury	8	8	8	24
Show 3, dance 4	Heather and Jonathan	Jive	*Can I Get A Witness*	Marvin Gaye	8	8	8	24
Show 3, dance 5	Apolo and Julianne	Jive	*You Never Can Tell*	Chuck Berry	7	8	8	23
Show 3, dance 6	Shandi and Brian	Jive	*Crocodile Rock*	Elton John	7	7	7	21
Show 3, dance 7	Laila and Maks	Tango	*Goldfinger*	Shirley Bassey	7	7	7	21
Show 3, dance 8	Billy Ray and Karina	Tango	*Rock The Casbah*	The Clash	7	7	7	21
Show 3, dance 9	John and Edyta	Tango	*Libertango*	Astor Piazzola	7	6	7	20
Show 3, dance 10	Clyde and Elena	Jive	*Bad Moon Rising*	Creedence Clearwater Revival	6	5	5	16
Show 3, dance 11	Maks, Karina, Brian, Elena, Jonathan, Cheryl, Alec, and Edyta	Artists/Dancers	*Eye of The Tiger*	Survivor				NONE
Show 3, dance 12	Tony, Julianne	Artists/Dancers	*So She Dances*	Josh Groban				NONE
Show 3, dance 13	Ciara's back up dancers	Artists/Dancers	*Like A Boy*	Ciara				NONE
Show 4, dance 1	Joey and Kym	Paso Doble	*Collecting The Ballots*	James Horner and Simon Rhodes	10	9	9	28
Show 4, dance 2	Apolo and Julianne	Waltz	*If You Don't Know Me By Now*	Simply Red	9	8	9	26
Show 4, dance 3	Ian and Cheryl	Waltz	*He Was Beautiful*	Shirley Bassey	7	9	8	24
Show 4, dance 4	Heather and Jonathan	Waltz	*Sandy's Song*	Dolly Parton	7	8	8	23
Show 4, dance 5	Laila and Maks	Paso Doble	*Les Toreadors*	Semyon Bychkov and Orchestre de Paris	7	7	7	21
Show 4, dance 6	Billy Ray and Karina	Paso Doble	*Black Betty*	Ram Jam	7	7	7	21
Show 4, dance 7	John and Edyta	Paso Doble	*It's A Kind Of Music*	Queen	6	5	5	16
Show 4, dance 8	Leeza and Tony	Paso Doble	*You Give Love A Bad Name*	Bon Jovi	6	5	5	16
Show 4, dance 9	Clyde and Elena	Waltz	*Foolish*	Johnny Cash	6	4	5	15

SEASON/SHOW/ DANCE NO	COUPLE	DANCE	SONG	ARTIST	JUDGE'S SCORES			
Show 4, dance 10	US Latin Champs: Andrei Gavriline and Elena Kryuchkova	Artists/Dancers	You'll Be Mine (Party Time)	Gloria Estefan				NONE
Show 4, dance 11	Brian and Julianne	Artists/Dancers	Lost in This Moment	Big & Rich				NONE
Show 4, dance 12	Tony and Cheryl, Alec and Edyta, and Drew Lachey	Artists/Dancers	Save a Horse, Ride A Cowboy	Big & Rich				NONE
Show 5, dance 1	Apolo and Julianne	Samba	I Like To Move It	Reel 2 Real	10	10	10	30
Show 5, dance 2	Laila and Maks	Rumba	Put Your Records On	Corinne Bailey Rae	9	10	9	28
Show 5, dance 3	Joey and Kym	Rumba	Besame Mucho	João Gilberto	8	8	9	25
Show 5, dance 4	Ian and Cheryl	Samba	Dance Like This	Wyclef Jean feat. Cludette Ortiz	8	8	8	24
Show 5, dance 5	Heather and Jonathan	Samba	Heaven Must Be Missing An Angel	Tavares	7	7	7	21
Show 5, dance 6	John and Edyta	Samba	Love Is In The Air	John Paul Young	6	6	6	18
Show 5, dance 7	Billy Ray and Karina	Rumba	What's Love Go To Do With It	Tina Turner	6	6	5	17
Show 5, dance 8	Clyde and Elena	Rumba	What's Going On	Marvin Gaye	4	5	4	13
Show 5, dance 9	Lisa Rinna and Chicago Dancers	Artists/Dancers	Roxie	Chicago (the musical) cast				NONE
Show 5, dance 10	Pro Dancers	Artists/Dancers	Finally Made Me Happy	Macy Gray				NONE
Show 5, dance 11	Group - Louis, Julianne, Christian Perry, Cheryl, Brian and Annette Nicole, Alec and Edyta	Group Dances/Jive	Zoot Suit Riot	Cherry Poppin' Daddies				NONE
Show 6, dance 1	Laila and Maks	Cha-cha	Hold On I'm Coming	Sam & Dave	9	9	10	28
Show 6, dance 2	Apolo and Julianne	Rumba	Cool	Gwen Stefani	9	9	10	28
Show 6, dance 3	Joey and Kym	Samba	A Little Respect	Erasure	9	9	9	27
Show 6, dance 4	Ian and Cheryl	Paso Doble	Waiting For Tonight	Jennifer Lopez	8	8	8	24
Show 6, dance 5	Heather and Jonathan	Paso Doble	Don't Cry For Me Argentina	Evita	7	8	8	23
Show 6, dance 6	Billy Ray and Karina	Jive	I Love to Boogie	T. Rex	7	7	7	21
Show 6, dance 7	John and Edyta	Mambo	Mambo Swing	Big Bad Voodoo Daddy	7	6	6	19
Show 6, dance 8	Group Swing - Joey, Kym, Heather, Jonathan, John, Edyta, Laila, Maks, Billy Ray, Karina, Apolo, Julianne, Ian, Cheryl	Group	Rock This Town	Stray Cats				NONE
Show 6, dance 9	Tony and Elena, Julianne and Derek Hough	Artists/Dancers	Super Duper Love	Joss Stone				NONE
Show 6, dance 10	Pro Dancers	Artists/Dancers	Tell Me 'Bout It	Joss Stone				NONE
Show 7, dance 1	Laila and Maks	Quickstep	Part Time Lover	Stevie Wonder	10	9	10	29
Show 7, dance 2	Joey and Kym	Foxtrot	The Way You Make Me Feel	Paul Anka	10	9	10	29
Show 7, dance 3	Ian and Cheryl	Tango	Holding Out For A Hero	Bonnie Tyler	9	9	9	27
Show 7, dance 4	Apolo and Julianne	Foxtrot	Steppin' Out With My Baby	Dinah Shore	9	8	9	26
Show 7, dance 5	John and Edyta	Foxtrot	That's Life	Frank Sinatra	8	7	8	23
Show 7, dance 6	Billy Ray and Karina	Waltz	Play Me	Neil Diamond	5	6	6	17
Show 7, dance 7	Laila and Maks	Samba	Brazil	Johnny Mathis	10	10	10	30
Show 7, dance 8	Joey and Kym	Jive	Slippin' and Slidin'	Little Richard	10	10	10	30
Show 7, dance 9	Apolo and Julianne	Mambo	Dr. Beat	Gloria Estefan	9	9	10	28
Show 7, dance 10	Ian and Cheryl	Mambo	Gimme That Light	Sean Paul	9	9	9	27
Show 7, dance 11	John and Edyta	Rumba	Under Pressure	Queen	7	8	7	22
Show 7, dance 12	Billy Ray and Karina	Samba	Living In America	James Brown	7	7	7	21
Show 7, dance 13	Pro Ballroom Kids,	Artists/Dancers	Boogie Shoes	KC & The Sunshine Band				
Show 7, dance 14	Jonathan Wilkins and Katusha Demidova	Artists/Dancers	Cry Over Me	Meatloaf				NONE
Show 7, dance 15	Louis, Cheryl, Brian, Kym, Alec, and Elena	Artists/Dancers	Bat Out of Hell	Meatloaf				NONE
Show 8, dance 1	Apolo and Julianne	Paso Doble	Carnaval de Paris	Dario G	10	8	10	28
Show 8, dance 2	Laila and Maks	Waltz	May Each Day	Andy Williams	9	9	9	27
Show 8, dance 3	Joey and Kym	Waltz	Always	Frank Sinatra	9	9	8	26
Show 8, dance 4	Ian and Cheryl	Foxtrot	Baby It's Cold Outside	Tom Jones	8	7	7	22
Show 8, dance 5	Billy Ray and Karina	Foxtrot	Stand By Your Man	Tammy Wynette	7	6	5	18
Show 8, dance 6	Apolo and Julianne	Tango	Jessie's Girl	Rick Springfield	10	10	10	28
Show 8, dance 7	Joey and Kym	Mambo	Pump It	Black Eyed Peas	10	9	10	29
Show 8, dance 8	Laila and Maks	Jive	Bad Bad Leroy Brown	Studio Group	9	8	9	26
Show 8, dance 9	Ian and Cheryl	Rumba	Imagine	John Lennon	8	8	9	25
Show 8, dance 10	Billy Ray and Karina	Mambo	My Way	Los Lonely Boys	6	7	7	20
Show 8, dance 11	Maks, Karina, Val Chmerkovskiy, and Valeriya Kazharinova	Artists/Dancers	Canned Heat	Jamiroquai				NONE

show results

SEASON/SHOW/ DANCE NO	COUPLE	DANCE	SONG	ARTIST	Carrie Ann Inaba	Len Goodman	Bruno Tonioli	Total
					JUDGE'S SCORES			
Show 8, dance 12	Tony and Elena	Artists/Dancers	*I'm Like a Bird*	Nelly Furtado				NONE
Show 8, dance 13	Louis and Cheryl	Artists/Dancers	*All Good Things*	Nelly Furtado				NONE
Show 9, dance 1	Apolo and Julianne	Quickstep	*Mr. Pinstripe Suit*	Big Bad Voodoo Daddy	10	10	10	30
Show 9, dance 2	Laila and Maks	Quickstep	*Walk Like An Egyptian*	The Bangles	10	10	10	30
Show 9, dance 3	Joey and Kym	Foxtrot	*My Guy*	Mary Wells	10	10	10	30
Show 9, dance 4	Ian and Cheryl	Tango	*Maneater*	Nelly Furtado	9	10	9	28
Show 9, dance 5	Laila and Maks	Cha-cha	*She's A Lady*	Tom Jones	10	10	10	30
Show 9, dance 6	Joey and Kym	Jive	*Jump Jive N' Wail*	Brian Seltzer Orchestra	10	10	10	30
Show 9, dance 7	Ian and Cheryl	Jive	*All Shook Up*	Elvis Presley	10	10	10	30
Show 9, dance 8	Apolo and Julianne	Cha-cha	*Push It*	Salt N' Pepa	10	9	10	29
Show 9, dance 9	Flamenco Dancing	Artists/Dancers	*Solea Mia*	Joaquin Cortez				NONE
Show 9, dance 10	Louis, Karina, Alec, and Edyta	Artists/Dancers	*Hero*	Enrique Iglesias				NONE
Show 9, dance 11	Pro Dancers	Artists/Dancers	*Do You Know*	Enrique Iglesias				NONE
Show 10, dance 1	Laila and Maks	Paso Doble	*Espana Cani*	Erich Kunzel	10	9	10	29
Show 10, dance 2	Apolo and Julianne	Paso Doble	*Carnaval de Paris*	Dario G	9	9	10	28
Show 10, dance 3	Joey and Kym	Tango	*Star Wars Cantina Band*	Meco	9	8	9	26
Show 10, dance 4	Apolo and Julianne	Freestyle	*Bust A Move*	Young MC	10	10	10	30
Show 10, dance 5	Joey and Kym	Freestyle	*Last Dance*	Donna Summer	10	10	10	30
Show 10, dance 6	Laila and Maks	Freestyle	*(Dance and Shout) Shake Your Body Down To The Ground*	Michael Jackson	9	8	9	26
Show 10, dance 7	Apolo and Julianne	Rumba	*Midnight Train To Georgia*	Gladys Knight	10	10	10	30
Show 10, dance 8	Joey and Kym	Cha-cha	*Groove Is In The Heart*	Deee-Lite	10	10	10	30
Show 10, dance 9	Paulina, Shandi, Leeza, Clyde	Group	*Too Darn Hot, Crocodile Rock, Independent Women, I Was Made To Love Her*	Various				NONE
Show 10, dance 10	Heather, John, Billy Ray, Ian	Group	*Mambo Italiano, Love Is In The Air, I Want My Mullet Back, All Shook Up*	Various				NONE
Show 10, dance 11	Alec, Karina, Edyta, Jonathan, Brian, Cheryl, Tony, Elena	Group	*It's Oh So Quiet*	Björk				NONE
Show 10, dance 12	All Couples	Group	*Everybody Dance*	Chic				NONE

Acknowledgments

The Authors wish to thank the following, whose kind contributions made this book possible:

The stars and professional dancers of *Dancing with the Stars,* Len Goodman, Carrie Ann Inaba, Bruno Tonioli, Tom Bergeron, Samantha Harris, Andrea Wong, John Saade, Conrad Green, Izzie Pick, Alex Rudzinski, Matilda Zoltowski, Rob Wade, Joe Sunkur, Michael Brooks, Toby Faulkner, Linda Giambrone, Melanie Mills, Mary Guerrero, Randall Christensen, Kirstin Gallo, Stephen Lee, Deena Katz, Vernon Chu, Jody Simon, Ian Moffitt, Brian Golby, Tara West, Sandy Mehlman, Andrea Andrade, Jeremy Whitham, Angie Meyer, Jared Paul, Harry Sandler. Chris Moore. All the people at ABC and Disney including, Melissa Harling, John Hanna, Carlos Williams, Bruce Gersh, Bob Miller, and Jean Marie Pierson. Our tireless editor Kathy Huck and everyone else at HarperCollins, Jane Friedman, Joe Tessitore, Angie Lee, Shelby Meizlik, Ellen Scordato and the Stonesong Press, Ruth Mannes, and Matthew Inman. Special thanks to our agents at ICM, Andrea Barzvi, Greg Lipstone and Lindsay Russell.

Lastly, none of this would be possible without all the fans who have made *Dancing with the Stars* the success it is.